"*Awake at 3 a.m.* is a necessary treatise for mothers with helpful insight and practical tools that offer the potential to soothe, ease, and nourish (something often directed at the newborn and not the mother herself). I wish this book existed during my pregnancy and my early experiences of motherhood. Suzannah Neufeld has truly offered us all a gift with her words of wisdom and expertise."

—Melanie Klein, Co-founder of the Yoga and Body Image Coalition and co-editor of *Yoga and Body Image*

"Suzannah Neufeld's experience as a psychotherapist and yoga therapist qualifies her to guide women through the sometimes rocky waters of pregnancy and new motherhood. But it is her personal honesty, her compassion, and her commitment to offer a light in dark waters that really makes this book stand out. *Awake at 3 a.m.* is a must have guide for all mamas."

—Jane Austin, Founder/Director Mama Tree Prenatal Yoga School and Director of Prenatal and Postnatal Program at Yoga Tree

"If you are pregnant or a new mom who is struggling, *Awake at 3 a.m.* is a map for the road to recovery. Neufeld's training, experience, and compassion oozes out of every page, leaving the reader feeling understood and supported. Her ability to bust through myths and debunk stereotypes, in particular about the practice of yoga, is incredibly powerful and effective. This book will change your life."

—Pec Indman, Chairperson of the Education and Training Committee, Postpartum Support International

"Suzannah Neufeld acknowledges and digs into all the feelings around parenting, no matter how messy they may be. In doing so, she shows us how yoga therapy can support new mothers and how motherhood can be embraced as a yogic practice."

—Roseanne Harvey, *It's All Yoga, Baby*

Awake at 3 a.m.

Yoga Therapy for Anxiety and Depression in
Pregnancy and Early Motherhood

SUZANNAH NEUFELD
MFT, C-IAYT

**PARALLAX
PRESS**

BERKELEY, CALIFORNIA

Parallax Press
P.O. Box 7355
Berkeley, California 94707
www.parallax.org

Parallax Press is the publishing division of Plum
Village Community of Engaged Buddhism, Inc.

Medical Disclaimer: The information in this book
is not intended or implied to be a substitute for
professional medical advice, diagnosis or treatment.
All content, including text, graphics, images, and
information contained in this book is for general
information purposes only.

Printed in the United States of America

Cover and text design by Debbie Berne
Cover illustration © Alexandra Bowman
Interior illustrations © Sara Christian
Author photo © Emily Gutman

ISBN: 978-1-941529-92-8

Library of Congress Cataloging-in-Publication Data is
available upon request.

1 2 3 4 5 / 22 21 20 19 18

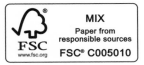

MIX
Paper from
responsible sources
FSC® C005010

To my husband, David, for being my 3 a.m. partner

Contents

Introduction 9

part one
the foundations

Difficult Experiences in Pregnancy and New Motherhood 24
Yoga Therapy: A Compassionate Mind-Body Response 42

part two
the practices

Section One
Make a Plan for Practice and for Support 58

Where do I begin? 59
You don't need a reason and it's not your fault 62
No, you won't "just be fine" 65
I'm not good at meditation 70
All you have to do is breathe 74
Affirmations are annoying 77
I never feel good anymore 81
I don't have time for yoga! 84
I'm having trouble bonding with my baby 87
Constant change is hard 90
I need help 94

Section Two
Welcome and Move with Your Thoughts and Feelings 99

I just want to feel better 100
Sadness 103
Anxiety, fear, and panic 107
I can't stop worrying! 110
Preoccupations 112
What if I can't stand this physical discomfort? 115
Rage 119
Sometimes I wonder if this was all a mistake 123
I should be grateful 126
Uncertainty 130
The darkest thoughts of depression 134

My baby won't stop crying 137
My baby has been up for hours and I can't sit down 140
Grief 143

Section Three
Cultivate Self-Compassion and Let Go of Comparisons 146

This is hard 147
How will I get through the rest of the day? 151
Compare and despair 154
Automatic negative thoughts 157
I'm not a good mom 160
I can't take any more advice! 163
The all-natural mandate 167
Body image blues 171
I need to make sure my baby is happy and healthy 175
What do they think of me? 178
I should . . . 181

Section Four
Develop Responsiveness and Flexibility 184

But I don't have any time to take care of myself! 185
Why didn't anyone tell me? 189
My body hurts 192
I'm hunched over all day 196
I'm so tired 199
I can't relax 203
No rest for the weary 206
A moment alone 210
Food struggles 214
Breastfeeding 218
Exercise 221
I can't handle this 226
Trauma 230
When maternal instincts don't kick in 233

Conclusion 237
Notes 239
Acknowledgments 241
Index 245

My images of myself in pregnancy and motherhood mostly take place in the light of the moon. I'm awake at 3 a.m., throwing up. I'm awake feeling the baby kick. I'm awake anxiously researching facts about baby health. I'm feeding my baby. I'm waking up to feed the baby again.

Night was always the hardest for me. In the day, with the sun shining, my demons vanished, love for my baby blossomed, work was meaningful, seeing friends brightened my mood. In the night, the unbearable sense that no one was coming to save me was overwhelming. I would think, *All I want to do is sleep. I am so desperate for sleep. I have never been this tired before. I can't do this. I want to be here for my baby. Why am I not a good enough mother to just do this?*

Becoming a parent is a blessing. Pregnancy is a miracle. My children are my favorite humans, teachers, and beloveds, and, in retrospect, they make those early nights of suffering infinitely worthwhile. I mean it with my whole heart (and only the slightest bit of irony) when I tell my daughters, "I love you to the moon and back."

But this is also true: being pregnant and having a baby are hard. Really hard. Even for the happiest mom on earth, it's certainly one of the greatest physical and endurance challenges that most of us have ever faced. It's a marathon of constant change and new, profound responsibility that you can't delegate elsewhere (though my greatest pregnant fantasy was making my husband carry the baby in *his* belly for me, even for just one trip around the grocery store). You are on the clock twenty-four hours a day. Add to that modern pressures to do it "perfectly"—wearing your baby all day, making your own baby food, taking adorable monthly photos and posting them online, and, of course, "bouncing back" to your pre-pregnancy body in just a few months.

For most moms, this combination of change in hormones and identity and the relentlessness of the physical demands of mothering bring difficult emotions and thoughts to the forefront. Sadness, rage, guilt, and anxiety may come to visit. You face the unknown, filling every day with fantasies and hopes—and worries, fears, and perhaps even terrors. For some moms, these feelings stay mild or manageable. Other moms, though, experience more intense emotional challenges, and develop depression or anxiety disorders.

Perinatal mood and anxiety disorders (PMADs) are the number one[1] "complication" of birth, affecting up to one in five new mothers. They can be serious, debilitating, and life-threatening. They affect not just moms who suffer, but also whole families that care about and rely on those moms. More than twice as many moms suffer from PMADs than gestational diabetes[2]. Yet while every mom is tested for diabetes, and robust support and treatment options exist for diabetes, moms who suffer emotionally are rarely acknowledged. Instead of receiving help, they are handed platitudes like "sleep when the baby sleeps," "let go of stress because it's bad for the baby," "just enjoy every minute because it goes by so fast," or "this too shall pass." This can be a lonely and confusing place to be—suffering profound fear, overwhelm, or sadness at a time when your friends and family expect you to be happy, radiant, and beatifically calm.

If this is you, you've picked up the right book. Above all, this book is meant to hold with compassion the challenge and exhaustion of this messy and transformative period in life. My intention is to help you make space for the darkness that can be so painful or scary to acknowledge.

These dark feelings can pose real, tangible difficulties for you and your family, so you likely picked up this book offering yoga therapy because you are looking for a solution. Many books or articles on yoga for moms have words like *calm* or *bliss* in the title and feature smiling, glowing, slim pregnant women on the cover. Yoga and mindfulness (and pregnancy in general!) in America are usually marketed as a path to fix all our woes, to make us happy, healthy, beautiful, loved, eternally youthful, sexy, peaceful, more productive, fully present. These promises sell well, because they prey on our attachments and reinforce our insecurities—again and again. But yoga doesn't actually work that way.

Yoga does offer effective coping skills for depression and anxiety, and this book will share these abundantly. Yoga doesn't, however, make us eternally calm or peaceful. It doesn't make us good mothers or turn our children into magical unicorns devoid of suffering. We are still exhausted. We still need sleep, food, care from our community or from professionals. Yoga doesn't fix us, but that's okay—even better than okay—because *we're not broken*. Yoga connects us to our whole self: mind, body, and heart. It connects us to our humanity and to our transcendent spaciousness. And when we hold our arms open to our full selves, welcoming even our darkness, we also welcome our light. We see the bigger picture of ourselves, remembering there is so much more to us than our struggles.

Yoga, like our newborn babies, wakes us up.

MY STORY

When I found out I was pregnant, I was so happy. I had normal fears about the possibility of miscarriage and about how my life was about to change, as well as some realistic knowledge that having experienced depression earlier in my life put me at risk for postpartum depression, but in general, my mood was optimistic and grateful. I felt like something magical was happening to me, and I almost thought I could see the "pregnancy glow" shimmering on my skin.

Everything changed a week later, when I started throwing up. For me, the term "morning sickness" felt like a cruel tease. I was not just nauseated in the morning. I was nauseated all day and all night. This was unrelenting, soul-crushing, tide-pulling-you-into-the-depths-of-the-ocean nausea. When I did throw up, I'd feel a few moments of relief, try to stand up, and then slowly feel the room start to spin—and it would start all over again. I would fall asleep in the bathroom, leaning on the toilet. It was hard to walk, move, breathe, smile. My regular yoga practice was out of the question.

After a few weeks of this, I began to feel helpless. In a total turn-around from the delight I had experienced just weeks before, I noticed that I had thoughts that my baby was like an alien parasite taking over my body and destroying me. When those thoughts would subside, and my love for my baby would come back, new thoughts would arise in which I would fear that something bad was going to happen to her because I was so sick.

In my desperate attempt to understand why this was happening to me, I would vacillate between fear, guilt, and rage. I blamed myself. I blamed my husband. I blamed my doctor. I blamed everyone I'd ever met. I felt angry that "no one told me that it could be like this." Other times, all this analysis fell away, and I fell into feral, desperate attacks of panic, and all I could think was, *I cannot take this anymore—I need to fix it NOW.*

I also felt deeply alone. I would listen to moms I knew say, "I know how that feels. I felt so sick when I was pregnant. Have you tried ginger? Totally worked for me." Yes—I had tried ginger! Here are all the other things I tried: acupuncture, vitamins, mint, sea bands, crackers, almonds, protein, grapes, apple cider vinegar, and any other suggestions friends, family, a random woman at a drug store, or Dr. Google had given me.

I went to a hypnotist who specialized in pregnancy. She told me that "morning sickness" is *always* a sign of feeling ambivalent about becoming a mother, and I could spend a few hundred bucks having her make me custom guided meditations to reduce my ambivalence and, thus, my nausea. At the time, I felt so ashamed and horrified by the thought that I might be ambivalent about becoming a mother. (Looking back, I wish I had said that any pregnant woman who denies feeling ambivalent is lying. You *should* feel ambivalent about becoming a mother—just like you would about any huge life change!)

I finally learned that I had a condition called *hyperemesis gravidarum*—extreme nausea and vomiting in pregnancy. This diagnosis led my doctor to prescribe a medication that I first took reluctantly and then gratefully. The medication mostly prevented me from getting sick, but there was still a baseline of nausea that made it impossible to enjoy life, plus occasional vomiting sprees that were hard to stop.

A vivid memory: At about ten weeks pregnant, once I'd been on the nausea medication for a few weeks, I was feeling okay for a few hours. I suggested to my husband that we take a slow walk to see some friends. We walked a few blocks and had a nice conversation. The sun was shining, and I felt the first crack of a smile on my face that I'd been able to muster in weeks. The smile felt foreign and distorted on my face, but real nonetheless. I felt enough hope to say out loud, "I think I may actually be starting to feel better. Maybe the worst of this is over." Five minutes later, I was throwing up in the street. A drunk guy walked out of a nearby bar, looked over, and said sympathetically, "Hey, sister, we've all been there."

In the taxi ride on the way home, I began to sob. I felt frustrated, hopeless, desperate, and scared. I just didn't know if I could make it through the rest of my pregnancy. Back at home in bed, I noticed my mind start to wish for death. I was terrified of these intrusive thoughts. *What kind of a pregnant woman thinks about wanting to die? What kind of a mother will I be? Why am I not more grateful? Will I ever recover from this? What will become of my baby and my marriage?*

Because I am a therapist, I realized quickly what was happening to me: I was experiencing acute prenatal depression and anxiety. I reached out for help from my husband, my friends, and my own therapist (yes, therapists go to therapy!). I began to draw on the tools I had used to cope in other dark times in my life to help me find my ground again.

At fifteen weeks pregnant, I talked myself into attending my first prenatal yoga class. Yoga was already a big part of my life—I had studied yoga for more than ten years and taught for six. The practice of yoga had guided me through difficult times before, and it seemed like the most familiar path for me to turn to for support. I just could not for the life of me imagine how I would bend myself into any physical postures without either throwing up or collapsing in fatigue.

I arrived at the studio and checked in with the teacher, Jane Austin, who had taught the basics of teaching pregnant students in my first yoga teacher training. "Hi," I said. "I'm not sure if you remember me—I was once in teacher training with you." And then I started to cry. I told her about how I hadn't been able to move much in the past three months and how awful I felt. I shared that being present in my body used to be a source of strength and calm, but lately it had just felt like misery and fear. I said I'd been curled up in a ball so much that I barely knew how to stand up straight again. Plus, my back had started to hurt, and I had a (literal) pain in my butt that might be sciatica.

Jane welcomed me with open arms and great compassion. She empathized with how awful I felt and didn't try to talk me out of my misery. She didn't promise it would get better. "I know!" she said, "It's so hard! It can feel impossible to move when you feel so awful." She told me that I wasn't alone, and that it was totally okay for me to show up at class curled up in a ball. She began to teach me, right there in the hallway, that yoga is a practice that can welcome us no matter what—that it can hold us when we feel physically sick, emotionally overloaded, and spiritually bereft.

Jane told me that it would be fine if I spent the entire class sitting or in a resting pose. She said I could try to do the poses and the movements and simply stop if it didn't feel right. She said listening to myself and taking care of myself was the most important part. She suggested that I start by just focusing on my breath and soaking in the experience of being in the room with other women going through some of the same things I was experiencing.

Then she taught me a breathing practice, *sitali pranayama*, which I could do if I felt nauseated. *Sitali* involves rolling your tongue up like a burrito. You inhale the air through the little circle you make with your tongue, and then close your mouth and breathe out through the nose. The air felt cold on my tongue as I breathed in, like ice cream on a hot day—sweet, delicious, and satisfying. I think it was the first moment of pure joy I had experienced since I'd gotten pregnant.

I went into the class, did a few downward dogs, cried a little, sat down for all the standing poses, and sitali'd till I could sitali no more. I practiced holding myself in my most tender, messy state. I began, slowly, to find my strength and resilience and to forge my new relationship with my daughter inside of me and my new identity as a mother.

Yoga wasn't and isn't a panacea. I don't remember the rest of that class, and I continued to feel awful for many weeks after that. Yoga didn't fix my nausea. It didn't even really help at all. But I felt compelled to go back, again and again, to be in that room, greeting and holding myself compassionately through all the discomforts, fears, and constant changes that pregnancy brought—mothering myself as practice for mothering my children. I began, also, to practice again at home. I changed my idea of what it meant to "do yoga." Previously, yoga for me had mostly involved doing vigorous movements and poses for exercise. Meditation, which I realized I had subconsciously relegated in my mind as "the boring part of yoga," now became its most essential element for me.

It's funny. Before I got pregnant, I assumed that being someone who does yoga, who eats "good" food and does "good" things, should exempt me from suffering. As if suffering were doled out according to merit. I thought pregnancy would make me calm, peaceful, strong, and wise, constantly connected to the sacred experience of growing a new soul, fully able to greet pain and change as "sensations" or primal experiences. I never would have guessed how much pregnancy would awaken me to the true power of yoga—not to fix, but to nourish, to hold, to accompany.

In the end, I didn't practice yoga or meditate because I thought I should, because I knew it was good for my baby, or even to fix myself—though the practice did slowly bring me a lot of healing. I practiced because yoga gave me something better.

Yoga became what I started to call my "well of sanity." In the darkest moments, it gave me access to awareness of my full self. Alongside my nausea, despair, and rumination, yoga helped me feel sensations in the parts of my body that didn't feel awful—my relaxed feet, my arms at ease. I could experience my breath as an unwavering companion. I could observe my distressed thoughts, watch them come, and watch them go.

Over and over, yoga helped me survive what my mind told me was unsurvivable. I turned to yoga and mindfulness as an act of desperation, a way to cope with the overwhelm, the heaviness, the darkness. But it cracked me open and put me in touch with the full messy beauty of what it means to be alive, to have created life, to care for a new soul. It transformed my struggle into a nourishing spiritual practice.

So when I'm up with my baby in the middle of the night, I'm awake at 3 a.m., and I'm also awake in another sense—*aware of how my mind works, how it creates despair. I'm awake to the needs, discomforts, and strength of my body. I'm awake to this baby, this here-for-just-one-second-and-then-growing-bigger baby, this sweet, warm, cuddly baby, this crying baby who needs me, who is human like me, who is part of this path of growth and suffering and love. I'm awake and aware of my breath, here, and here again, filling me up, soothing, energizing, connecting me.*

Each year of motherhood, I find new ways that yoga fortifies me for the sacred, beautiful, and unbelievably challenging job of being a mom. Reciprocally, motherhood deepened my yoga practice. Indeed, new motherhood is the perfect time to "awaken," since you will be forced to wake up many times a night!

MY APPROACH

The approach I offer in this book is based on yoga therapy, mindfulness and acceptance-based therapies, and self-compassion. The yoga therapy here isn't the fancy acrobatic yoga you see on the cover of a magazine. I won't even talk much about alignment in the poses (just enough to keep you safe). These are yoga practices for feeling from the inside, not performing for others. You won't need ninety minutes, an expensive mat, or any special clothes (though for me, half of the reason to practice yoga—or get pregnant—is getting to wear stretchy pants whenever you want). You won't need anything but yourself.

I share these practices from my heart—they were my balm, my comfort, my solace, my "well of sanity" during my own mood and anxiety struggles in pregnancy and new motherhood. I also share this approach from my knowledge and experience in the role of psychotherapist, pre- and postnatal yoga teacher, and yoga therapist working with pregnant and new moms.

I'll address the myths and misunderstandings that may prevent us from trying yoga therapy. These misunderstandings mirror some of the messages we moms have received that interfere with enjoying new motherhood:

- You must do things perfectly.
- You have to be good at something before you even know how to do it.
- Humans are good or bad, broken or fixed.
- Love can't exist alongside hate.
- Exhaustion can't exist alongside excitement.
- Sorrow somehow erases joy, and vice versa.
- If you accept yourself, you'll never grow and change.

I will cover how to realistically incorporate meditation, breathing, and movement practices into new motherhood. You will learn practices that welcome and address all kinds of difficult feelings. You will find practical, concrete tools you can immediately use in moments of desperation, when you encounter your darkest thoughts or urges.

You will also learn things you can say to yourself and those around you to ride out the waves of anxiety and depression with kindness and compassion.

HUMILITY

It is important from the start to say that this book is a humble attempt to convey the way that I've understood yoga and how it helps me and the women around me. Yoga is not mine—none of what is written here has been invented by me or belongs to me. Yoga is a deep and complex philosophy and science that originates in India. I am a white Jewish woman who lives in California. I've practiced for only sixteen years—I am and will always be a beginner.

Similarly, while I have had my own experiences with motherhood and perinatal mood difficulties, and have listened to many others in their experiences, I only humbly approach the challenge of detailing the infinitely unique forms of suffering that mothers experience and how they heal. Tolstoy famously began his novel *Anna Karenina* with the words, "All happy families are alike, each unhappy family is unhappy in its own way.[3]" Such is the truth for mothers struggling in pregnancy and postpartum.

Some moms experience anxiety, some depression, some anger or rage. Some have difficulty bonding with their babies, and some just feel very alone. Some have struggled with their moods throughout their lives; for others, pregnancy and postpartum is the first time they have felt this way. Some moms have gone through losses or infertility, some have many children, some just one. I am sure I will leave the experiences of some out, and you will find things in here that miss the boat for you or that do not resonate with you. I hope you will find something in here that does resonate, and that helps you on your healing journey.

I also know that the styles and particular struggles of mothering I describe in this book are localized in the community and time I live in—I live in the Bay Area, where right now there is a culture of intensity and perfectionism in parenting that affects most of the moms I know, both high- and low-income, whether they accept it or reject it. We are expected to do everything we can to create perfectly happy, smart, healthy kids—often at our own expense. We also do so in relative isolation—often dealing with newborns, a full-time job, and older kids with no family around to support us. If you live elsewhere, you may not relate to all of this, and perhaps there are other pressures or expectations in your own community.

Financial instability is another huge and real stressor for many new mothers. Many moms cannot afford a yoga class, and many work long hours to support their families, leaving little time for self-care. Accordingly, this book focuses entirely on practices that can be practiced for free, and that you can do with your baby or while at work.

We are also in a time of growing awareness about gender, and indeed what it means to call oneself a mother or a woman. I write from my personal experience of womanhood and the largely cisgender female population of clients and students I have worked with. I want to acknowledge that there are mothers who do not go through pregnancy or childbirth, and transgender men and nonbinary people who have babies. I hope that this book will offer practices that would be useful for all new parents—including fathers and adoptive parents, who can also suffer from PMADs.

HOW TO USE THIS BOOK

Part 1 of this book, "The Foundations," lays the groundwork. Chapter 1 begins with a thorough exploration of the ways we can suffer in pregnancy and new motherhood and offers a deeper understanding of clinical perinatal mood and anxiety disorders. Chapter 2 explores this new approach of yoga therapy, addressing how and why we might begin or re-engage with a yoga practice at a time when energetic resources are low and our efforts are dedicated in service of these new little lives that need such care and protection.

Part 2, "The Practices," is broken down into fifty chapters—each one related to a particular way that you might be suffering or struggling, and describing a yoga practice or two that could offer skills to face it.

The fifty chapters are organized into four sections, fleshing out what I would call the four essential aspects of a yoga therapy approach to the postpartum period:

1   Make a plan for practice and support
2   Welcome and move with your thoughts and feelings
3   Cultivate self-compassion and let go of comparisons
4   Develop responsiveness and flexibility

You can read the chapters in any order, or just read those that speak to you. This book is meant to fit into your very busy life, to be read when you are exhausted and multitasking.

INTENTION

I know you are tired and overworked, and what you do not need is yet another thing to do or fix. I offer this book in the hopes that you see that yoga is not a way to improve or perfect yourself as a mother or as a person, or a secret to engineering a happy, perfect child with a high IQ, inspiring grit, and dauntless self-confidence.

I hope to cut through all these expectations, agendas, and attachments, and give you tools to take a moment, just a moment, to just enjoy how your baby smells right now. To survive feeling depressed and anxious with your baby in the middle of the night. To give you one practice in this culture that is not about being right, good, or happy, and is just about being. My hope is that the book will let you off the hook a little, let you breathe a bit easier, and give you some options for practices that might feel nourishing to your heart.

Mothers heal from depression and anxiety every day. Working with new moms is deeply rewarding as a therapist. I see them heal slowly but surely. I see moms rediscover themselves, integrating their new identities, building new community. Babies become less demanding, they learn to talk and offer love back, and families find their footing. The middle-of-the-night wake-ups eventually become a memory. I have all the faith in the world that you can heal from PMADs, and I hope this book makes that process a more meaningful one.

Last—in writing a book about how mothers can use yoga to alleviate their own suffering, I run a danger of communicating the idea that the suffering of mothers is our own fault and only our own responsibility. It's important to say that much pain emanates from the lack of support women too often experience in our society. Sexism, racism, and systematic poverty create situations where many do not have resources for basic self-care, and where trauma complicates any attempt at healing.

In the face of these injustices, it pains me to hear people say that yoga teaches us that our reactions are all that matter or that if we focus on our own equanimity, we can free ourselves of all suffering. This turns yoga into something that puts us back to sleep, that makes us more amenable to societal injustice.

Yoga at its core is about liberation, and it is a hollow liberation if we do not use the freedom and perspective it gives us to engage meaningfully with the world around us. My hope is that we can, over time, use the strength we each draw from our own healing to lift up mothers around us and to fight together against societal forms of neglect, ignorance, and oppression.

part one

The Foundations

Difficult Experiences in Pregnancy and New Motherhood

Having a baby is usually thought of as the most joyful, blissful time in one's life. We believe that pregnant women glow, take pictures of adorable new babies, fawn over their tiny clothing. For many new mothers, however, the early days of pregnancy and parenthood are marked by a struggle with blue moods and anxious thoughts. Hormonal shifts, sleep deprivation, the shock of a major lifestyle and identity change, and this culture's lack of support for new families make pregnant and new mamas vulnerable to challenging emotions and states of mind.

Additionally, parents in today's world experience unprecedented pressure. We are expected to raise the "Happiest Baby on the Block," who will be organically fed, safe and protected but not helicopter-parented, attached but not needy, self-confident but not selfish. We are not supposed to stress out about any of this because stress hurts our kids and we need to learn to relax. We are supposed to do this all naturally, without the help and guidance of our families and communities. We are supposed to do this all with little to no paid parental leave, no subsidized childcare, and little-to-no mental health care coverage. And then we are supposed to post pictures of ourselves and our families smiling through it all on social media. #blessed.

Often, moms feel shock or self-criticism when we realize that pregnancy or new motherhood is also hard. You expect to feel like a goddess and have a "maternal instinct" kick in. Then you start to feel uncomfortable in your body, have terrible heartburn, and miss the life you had before you got pregnant. You miss your beer, or sushi, or your ability to focus at work, or making it through a movie without having to pee. You miss your sex life. Or you don't miss your sex life—and feel guilty about that. Or your new baby cries all night long and you can't figure out what they need. Or you expected to get back to your pre-pregnancy weight and didn't realize you would still be rocking maternity pants a few months later. Or an older woman at the supermarket coos over the baby and tells you to "cherish every moment because they grow up so fast" and you sink into shame. Just that morning, you were wishing your baby would go the f*** to sleep! You wonder: *What is wrong with me? Why am I failing at motherhood?*

Many moms who do not suffer from a clinical mood or anxiety challenge have a hard time during pregnancy and new motherhood. You may struggle with a fear of birth, the pressure to be a perfect mother, our society's unattainable body image expectations, the unreasonable sleep deprivation involved in having a newborn, and the Sisyphean tasks of feeding, burping, changing, and rocking over and over and over.

This book is meant to support all moms who have feelings of over-whelm, stress, and exhaustion. However, if you are picking this up, it is likely that you might have a clinical diagnosis of a perinatal mood or anxiety disorder (PMADs). While I don't want clinical terms to make you feel pigeonholed or pathologized, I do think understanding these conditions can be helpful. They may provide you with validation or guidelines for treatment, or help communicate to your care providers or family members what you think is going on with you.

Suffering mothers often think that their suffering is normal and to be expected, or that they are only having a hard time because they are somehow inherently bad or deficient. Often, they don't recognize symptoms of PMADs because of stereotypes they have about it. For that reason, I want to spend some time going over the clinical defini-tions of PMADs.

PERINATAL MOOD AND ANXIETY DISORDERS (PMADs)

Baby blues is the most common type of mood challenge experienced by new parents. Baby blues, which is a clinical term, begin in the first week after birth and last for a few days or a few weeks. They are characterized by mild mood swings and are normal—50 to 80 percent of new mothers report some symptoms of baby blues.[4] If a few days after childbirth you find yourself crying for no reason, snapping at your partner for changing a diaper the wrong way, or panicking briefly about whether your baby is still breathing, you might have the baby blues.

The symptoms of baby blues are similar to those of PMADs, but are marked by a difference in when they happen, how long they last, and how intense they are. While baby blues happen in the first few weeks of motherhood, PMADs can happen any time during pregnancy or the first year after childbirth, and affect about 20 percent of mothers[5]. PMADs last longer—sometimes even beyond the first year. The symptoms are more severe and yet sometimes less obvious than an episode of crying. They affect feelings, thoughts, and behaviors. PMADs can also affect women who have experienced pregnancy loss, abortion, or adoption. Partners, including men, also experience PMADs, though less frequently.

You've probably heard of PMADs by the name *postpartum depression,* or even just "postpartum." Postpartum depression is a misnomer in a couple of ways: PMADs don't just happen in the postpartum period, and they aren't just depression. We use the word *perinatal* instead because it refers to the entire time period of pregnancy and new motherhood. Mood and anxiety problems don't hit moms only after birth. Many moms who have PMADs experience an onset of symptoms while pregnant. Setting up and getting treatment while pregnant can be immensely helpful for making the postpartum period more manageable.

Instead of talking only about perinatal depression, most therapists and doctors now talk about perinatal "mood and anxiety" disorders. This is because the word *depression* paints a picture of a fairly homogenous form of suffering. We picture a sad new mom, crying in bed. PMADs can look like this, but many new moms have very different symptoms. So many moms suffer from anxiety and panic while pregnant and never ask for help because they only know about postpartum depression. They might say, "I don't feel sad at all, and I'm very bonded with my baby, I just can't sleep because I'm so worried all the time."

If you are suffering, check out the list of symptoms below. Some may seem familiar to you; some may seem foreign. You don't need to have them all to have PMADs—even one symptom deserves support.

Symptoms of PMADs *can* include:

Feelings

- Sadness
- Guilt or shame
- Overwhelm or dread
- Irritability or rage
- Anxiety, fear, or panic
- Numbness
- Loss of joy or pleasure
- Lack of interest, connection, or love
- Physical discomfort like headaches, exhaustion, or pain

Thoughts

- Thoughts like: *I'm not a good enough mom. All the other moms are better. My child/partner/friend/job deserves better than me. Maybe this was a mistake. I can't do this. It just doesn't come naturally to me.*
- Thoughts about something bad happening to you or your baby
- Constant worries
- Preoccupations with your health or your baby's health
- During pregnancy, fears and worries about birth and pain
- Thoughts of suicide, homicide, or wanting to die

- Intrusive memories of past events or previous experiences of giving birth

Behaviors

- Crying a lot
- Problems with sleep or appetite (too much or too little)
- Difficulty asking for help or allowing others to help with the baby
- Difficulty bonding or connecting with the baby
- Compulsive cleaning and checking on baby, home, or health
- Compulsively reading baby/parenting books or researching on the Internet
- Avoidance of feared situations like being alone with baby, leaving baby with others, or bringing baby out in public
- Use and abuse of alcohol or other drugs

Let's talk a little more about specific subtypes of PMADs.

Perinatal Depression

When we hear the word *depression*, we may think, *Oh—this is just a bad mood.* Nope: clinical depression is different from the everyday sadness that people often call "feeling depressed." Sadness usually makes sense in response to loss, conflict, or pain in your life. This emotion may even be a useful sign that you need to make some changes in your relationships or your job, or that your soul is in need of some care.

Major depression, on the other hand, gives rise to a devastating sense of hopelessness, worthlessness, and despair that prevents change rather than inspiring it. With clinical depression, you may lose your ability to feel joy, to connect with loved ones, and to imagine a better future. People with depression often think about death or running away as a form of escape. When you have depression, you are likely to criticize and blame yourself constantly. Alternately, you may criticize and blame others. This anger often then doubles back on to yourself, bringing feelings of shame and guilt for angry outbursts. Rage and irritability toward your loved ones are common, but often missed, signs of perinatal depression.

Depression can range from mild to severe. You may be able to function normally without anyone knowing you have depression. When it is stronger, engaging in tasks of daily living can feel nearly impossible, and functioning can be greatly affected. Depression often carries thoughts of suicide or wanting to die, and thus is not to be taken lightly—it can be a life-threatening condition. Too many moms have taken their lives when suffering from untreated perinatal depression.

Perinatal Bipolar Disorder

Most people who suffer from perinatal bipolar disorder also experienced bipolar disorder before becoming pregnant. With bipolar disorder, you experience periods of major depression and periods of what is called *mania* (or *hypomania*, a milder version). In mania, you may feel awake, motivated, excited, creative, or agitated. You may want to stay up all night long working on projects, or feel invincible, like you do not need a break at all. Bipolar episodes are often triggered by unstable sleep patterns, making the postpartum period one of the times someone with bipolar disorder is most vulnerable. Perinatal bipolar disorder may also lead to perinatal psychosis.

Perinatal Anxiety

Perinatal anxiety disorders may be the most under-recognized PMADs because the symptoms can look so much like a typical concerned and caring mom, and because you may not feel sad or down at all. Moms with anxiety disorders worry about their babies so much that they struggle to enjoy themselves or be present. Anxiety may be generalized, so worry attaches itself to whatever is going on. Moms may worry what friends think of them, if they are taking good enough care of their baby, if the laundry is folded right. They may worry about their jobs, politics, and the environment. The list is endless.

Moms with anxiety may have trouble slowing down and resting. Anxiety is sometimes most recognizable as physical concerns—feeling dizzy, shaky, or out of breath. Another common sign of perinatal anxiety is difficulty falling or staying asleep.

Moms with anxiety may also have panic attacks, where they feel they cannot breathe, or feel like they're going to throw up, or like they're going crazy. Sometimes fear of having a panic attack can lead to being afraid to leave the house or to be left alone.

Perinatal Obsessive-Compulsive Disorder (OCD)

OCD is a disorder in which the person becomes stuck on certain thoughts, images, or urges known as obsessions. Just as with generalized anxiety disorder, obsessions can be tricky to diagnose because they may look like the same worries that many moms share. Maybe you are nervous about your baby being exposed to chemicals or germs or afraid of SIDS (sudden infant death syndrome). Maybe you worry that you would accidentally hurt your baby. These are normal things to worry about! Without OCD, you know these are passing thoughts that will likely not come true, and you move on to thinking about other things. With OCD, however, the worries get very sticky in your mind and feel intrusive. Moms with OCD can't stop thinking these thoughts.

With OCD, you then engage in compulsive behaviors or mental acts to try and get the worries to go away—cleaning constantly, having the house checked for chemicals, getting blood tests, replaying your day over and over in your mind, or asking repeatedly for reassurance from your partner. In pregnancy, you may get an at-home heart monitor and check the baby's heart rate over and over again. You may feel compelled to spend hours online doing research on various conditions that could befall your baby. These compulsive behaviors seem to provide comfort in the moment, perhaps a sense of control, but then the anxiety returns and the urge to perform these behaviors comes back. In addition to these active compulsions, you may have avoidance compulsions, meaning you feel a need to avoid places and experiences to keep the obsessions and fears at bay.

Some OCD compulsions look like they make sense: cleaning and checking, for instance. You might struggle to see them as something unhelpful. Some make less sense, and the urges can be frustrating— for example, a need to think certain thoughts in a certain order, or tap certain things, or count the number of times you do things in order to ward off harming your baby. Moms with these kinds of compulsions are more likely to realize something is up.

One of the most difficult of OCD symptoms that moms can experience is the fear that they are going to harm their baby. Moms may have painful thoughts and mental images of hurting, dropping, abandoning, or even molesting their baby. With OCD, the mom will experience a great deal of shame about these thoughts and believe that just because she had the thought, she is a bad mother who is planning to actually carry that behavior out. This mom may engage in all sorts of rituals to keep herself from having these thoughts. She may also compulsively avoid spending time with her baby, in order to protect the baby.

Post-Traumatic Stress Disorder (PTSD)

Perinatal PTSD can be triggered by fertility problems, miscarriages, past baby loss, illness during pregnancy, traumatic birth, or a sick baby that needs to spend time in the NICU (neonatal intensive care unit). Trauma is defined as an experience of witnessing or being exposed to threats such as death or injury to yourself or a loved one. Trauma can often lead to hypervigilance—feeling overly alert to danger and having your fight-or-flight system on overdrive. It can lead to replaying over and over in your mind what happened, even after others tell you that you should be "over it." It can lead to a sense of numbness, of psychologically leaving your body or your situation throughout the day, whenever something triggers a memory of the trauma. These are all adaptive responses your body and mind make to prevent something bad from happening again, but they make it hard to be present in your life now, when you are safe.

If you have trauma from other circumstances in your life, like abuse or neglect in your childhood or teen years, this too can come up again in pregnancy or postpartum. You might worry about how to protect your baby so that nothing bad ever happens to them like it did to you. If you were neglected emotionally or physically by your own parents or caregivers, you might feel a resurgence of hurt or anger about the neglect, as you put so much time and energy into caring for your own child.

Perinatal Eating Disorders

Eating disorders are not technically mood or anxiety disorders, but they seemed important to include here because they are likely to develop, re-emerge after a period of recovery, or worsen at times in life when hormones are changing—during puberty, pregnancy, postpartum, and menopause. Appetite changes, shape changes, and confusing messages about food and weight gain abound. Well-meaning care providers issue warnings about both not gaining enough weight and gaining too much weight.

Moms with eating disorders may restrict food intake, overeat or binge eat, or purge calories consumed by throwing up, fasting, or over-exercising. Exhaustion and focus on care for a baby make it hard to listen to hunger and fullness signals. Food can become a way to cope, to find comfort, and to punish yourself. You may find yourself obsessively focused on changes in your body and weight in pregnancy. The focus on thinness, youth, and return to a pre-baby body means that most all moms in our culture struggle with how they feel about their bodies, even if they don't have eating disorders. Body image difficulties can certainly contribute to depression and feelings of shame and worthlessness.

One less obvious way that an eating disorder may show up during pregnancy is in obsessive focus on eating only healthy, "clean" food. You may have good intentions about taking perfect care of your baby, but when this focus becomes extreme, you may not be able to eat with others, limiting your social support, or you may not be able to get enough food to nourish yourself and your baby adequately.

Perinatal Psychosis

Perinatal psychosis is a rare form of PMADs, occurring in about one out of a thousand births, but it is often the condition that gets the most media attention because it can have grave consequences. Psychosis involves a break from reality. People with psychosis may have hallucinations—hearing or seeing things that are not there—or have delusional beliefs about themselves, their babies, or their loved ones. When perinatal psychosis occurs, it often happens right after birth, and can be accompanied by not sleeping for days. Psychosis is a very serious condition, and requires immediate and intensive medical support.

RISK FACTORS

If you feel shame or guilt over a diagnosis of PMADs, I encourage you to hold yourself gently around that, too. PMADs are not your fault! PMADs don't happen to people because they are weak or bad mothers. They are caused by a myriad of factors—genetic, biological, personal, and societal. Scientists have linked mood and anxiety disorders to genes and to changes in neurotransmitters in the brain, such as serotonin and dopamine. Sensitivity to hormones such as cortisol, estrogen, and oxytocin are implicated, too. Psychologists tie PMADs to life events, thought patterns, loss, poverty, and early childhood attachments. Risk factors include the following:

- Personal or family history of depression/anxiety
- Depression/anxiety during pregnancy
- History of severe PMS
- History of miscarriage or baby loss
- History of fertility problems or treatment
- Traumatic birth
- Baby care stress: colic, baby health problems, baby in the NICU
- Social isolation
- Inadequate support in caring for baby
- Major stressors: financial, marital, loss, change in occupation, moving
- Current or past domestic violence, trauma, or poverty

You may have heard the expression "canary in the coal mine." In the old days, coal miners would bring canaries with them down to work in the mines. If the mine was letting off toxic gas, the canaries would be affected before the miners. A canary's tiny lungs are more vulnerable than a human's lungs, and when the poor creatures became ill or died, the miners would know that their environment was not safe, and would leave quickly.

Mothers with perinatal mood and anxiety disorders are a bit like those canaries in the coal mine. They have vulnerability, due to individual risk factors, to the poisonous way that our society treats mothers. Just as the canaries were not sick before going into the coal mines, moms with PMADs are not inherently sick or weak, and they are not just "dealing badly" with something that is fine for everyone else. The way our society treats moms and families affects everyone eventually.

Our society does not adequately take care of mothers. We do not fund Planned Parenthood, to allow mothers to have choice in becoming a mother. And once babies are born, we offer more care to the babies than to the mothers. Babies get frequent pediatric visits in the first few weeks of life. Moms get one appointment. And that's if they are lucky enough to have health insurance. Even with insurance, mental health coverage is scant and expensive.

We live isolated lives. Moms are expected to have a baby and then be up and at it the next day. Outside of specific cultural groups, we do very little in the way of offering a new family care and support. Most of our traditions of showing a new family support are focused on offering material things—buying cute baby clothes, receiving blankets, and piles of gadgets. A family might receive a casserole or two in the week the baby comes home, but after that, most moms have to cook for themselves. We do not offer moms adequate paid parental leave. We do not offer partners adequate paid parental leave, which usually leaves the bulk of the work of childcare and home care on mothers. We offer no free, state-sponsored or community-offered childcare. We offer no easy path to finding and choosing reliable childcare, even if you can afford it.

We doubly let down moms of color, moms with fewer resources, and immigrant moms, who are much more likely to lack services and support—and, correspondingly, to suffer from PMADs.

We talk a lot in our culture about the importance of self-care, and you'll see a lot of that in this book. But while focus on self-care is important, this cultural tide also sends a message to moms that the community is not planning to care for you. My hope is that we can keep developing ways for our community to change and offer proactive care for moms. These changes will have to happen on both local and grander political stages.

TREATMENT FOR PMADs

The risk factors and causes of PMADs are so complex that a solid plan of healing will need to address you as a whole person as well as address the community around you. If you suspect you may be experiencing PMADs, ask for professional support as soon as possible. PMADs respond well to early treatment, and untreated PMADs often get worse.

Conventional Treatment for PMADs

The professions of psychiatry and psychotherapy have developed a multitude of effective ways to support moms with PMADs. Traditionally, any form of clinical depression or anxiety was treated with psychodynamic therapy, also known as the talking cure. Psychodynamic therapy hypothesizes that current psychological pain is caused by unconscious defense mechanisms, responses to early childhood experiences, and altered childhood development. In therapy sessions, patients speak aloud what they think and feel, over time "making the unconscious conscious." This process aims to enable the patient to live their lives in a freer, more creative, more connected, and less defended manner.

In the last fifty years, cognitive and behavioral approaches have also become commonly used to treat depression and anxiety. In general, cognitive behavioral therapy (CBT) posits that most psychological problems can be connected to faulty cognitions (thoughts) and unhelpful behaviors that maintain these faulty cognitions. CBT involves examining your thoughts, beliefs, and behaviors, and encourages you to choose and practice more helpful ones. If avoidance is a problem, systematic exposure to feared experiences is encouraged. Behaviors that promote health, such as practicing relaxation and building supportive community, are also often part of CBT. Among conventional treatments for anxiety and depression, CBT is the one with the most scientific evidence to support its effectiveness.

Recently, mainstream psychotherapy has begun to notice that the earlier approaches left something missing—mindfulness! Dialectical behavior therapy (DBT) and Acceptance and Commitment Therapy (ACT) are now widely used and researched approaches to therapy, and both borrow heavily from Eastern mindfulness traditions. These approaches still encourage changing behavior, as in CBT, but shift away from trying to change thoughts.

Mindful therapies teach us that thoughts, including painful ones, arise whether we want them to or not. Trying to change or control thoughts can be an impossible struggle—just another thing at which we feel we are failing. Instead, these approaches promote the practice of noticing and accepting thoughts without judging or attaching to them. In mindfulness-based therapy, you learn to see thoughts and feelings as passing events and choose behaviors based on your unchanging values and wisdom. Practices such as meditation are encouraged in order to develop a more compassionate and collaborative relationship with yourself.

In any form of psychotherapy for PMADs, you will likely develop a relationship with a provider who is caring and warm, offering compassion, wisdom, expertise, connection, and an open-minded, non-judgmental ear. You will strategize and problem-solve in order to improve sleep, nutrition, and relationships—all key pieces of healing. You will explore how to balance your care for your baby and yourself. Couples therapy is often indicated, both because one's partner can be the greatest source of support and because PMADs can be so confusing and painful to the relationship.

Support groups are another common therapeutic outlet for moms with PMADs. New moms need validation, connection, and compassion, and groups of other new moms are a great place to find it. Some groups are led by therapists and some are peer-led. Some are focused specifically on moms with PMADs and some on support for all moms through this challenging time.

Psychiatry adds to the tools provided by psychotherapy by addressing imbalances in brain chemistry. For a mom with severe depression or anxiety, psychotherapy alone is often not enough to improve her symptoms. She may be so depressed or anxious that she cannot engage well in psychotherapy or even begin to consider adding in what you may think of as forms of "natural" healing like yoga, meditation, or social engagement.

Medication for depression is often derided in the holistic health community as taking the easy way out or "just medicating." Antidepressants are flippantly referred to as "happy pills." This rhetoric is dangerous, as it creates shame, spreads ignorance, and puts up barriers to these treatments that can be lifesaving. A more balanced view of psychiatric medication understands that these drugs will not cure depression on their own, nor will they prevent healing from happening through "natural" means. At best, antidepressants will give you the energy and support you need to effectively show up for and benefit from supportive community, psychotherapy, and yoga.

Moms often tell me that they have assumed or been told that you cannot or should not take psychiatric medications while pregnant or nursing. This is not true. There are some medications that doctors will feel very comfortable prescribing, and together you can talk about and examine the risks and benefits, helping you make an informed decision that is right for you.

Many moms I see worry about taking medication, even after a doctor recommends it. They worry about birth defects, autism, or effects on their child's intelligence or behavior in the future. They feel like they're in a bind because they believe having PMADs isn't good for their baby *and* they believe medications aren't good for their baby. Every mom wants her baby to be healthy and live their best life. And what a double wound—the pain that she is suffering from having depression or anxiety, and then the pain of the guilt, shame, or fear about what it means for her baby. This is often where the thought *I'm a terrible mom* begins.

Reassurance doesn't usually help much—because how could a therapist say, "Your child will be fine!" Of course there is always the possibility, even likelihood, that your child, like every human that came before, will have struggles in life, whether or not you have PMADs or take medication. That said, I think it is important to hold a more nuanced perspective.

Yes, some studies have shown that there are possible small risks to taking medication. However, studies have also shown that untreated maternal depression is a risk, too. PMADs can be life-threatening to the mom—and thus harmful to her baby. PMADs might mean you aren't able to eat, sleep, or care for yourself optimally, which also affects a growing baby. Moms with PMADs are more likely to turn to alcohol and other drugs that definitely affect babies. The risks to the baby of untreated maternal depression are often greater than the risks of taking medication. Stopping medication right before pregnancy, or mid-pregnancy, greatly increases the risk and severity of PMADs.

Similarly, you may have assumed or been told that if you do take medication, you should take the smallest dose. While this line of thinking has some logic to it, this is not, unfortunately, the way meds work. If you take a medication at so small a dose that it is ineffective, your baby is then exposed to both the medication *and* PMADs. And then you might feel guilty for both struggling to be present with your baby and taking medication. Most importantly, if you are under-medicated, the medication may not help you enough—and you deserve all the help you need.

The good news is that no matter what, your baby is not doomed. There are many things you can do to protect and care for your child now and in the future—we will cover many of them in this book. PMADs are treatable, and getting treatment helps both you and your baby.

If possible, I strongly recommend you see a psychiatrist who specializes in PMADs, as opposed to an obstetrician or primary care physician. You'll want a sensitive, supportive specialist who is up to date on what medications and doses are safest and most effective.

Because there are many forms of treatment available, don't think you have to stick with the first one offered to you. Every mother is different. If you aren't feeling better with the first approach, therapist, doctor, support group, or medication you try, advocate for yourself—even when it's scary or a provider balks—and ask for help that better suits your needs. Most moms need to diversify, supporting themselves in more than one way, perhaps complementing conventional treatments with mind-body approaches.

Complementary Treatments for PMADs

Forms of complementary support that many moms with PMADs find helpful include postpartum doula care, acupuncture, chiropractic care, herbal medicine, nutritional support, and massage/bodywork. Many of these approaches are called "mind-body" approaches because they treat and care for a mom with PMADs as a whole person.

Yoga therapy is a rich, holistic mind-body approach encompassing mindfulness, movement, and the wisdom of a compassionate attitude. Prenatal and postnatal yoga classes are accessible in many US communities and online, and offer moms with PMADs an opportunity to connect with other mothers. Yoga often feels less stigmatizing or intimidating for moms than other approaches because yoga is something they are familiar with and might have experienced as healing at other times in their lives. Yoga therapy can be a cost-effective and time-effective approach. Even if you see a professional yoga therapist, you are given tools that you can practice at home for free, with a baby in arms.

Yoga therapy also supports and enriches so much of what conventional treatments have to offer. As both a conventional talk psychotherapist and a yoga therapist, I notice every day the parallels and connections in the healing work my clients do. In both approaches we:

- Make the unconscious conscious: increase our awareness of our deepest truths and deepest selves
- Free up stuck energy
- Notice unhelpful thoughts
- Practice kindness and compassion toward self
- Practice mindfulness
- Use the body as a source of healing—promoting rest, sleep, nutrition, exercise/movement
- Believe in a person's inherent strength and promote hope for healing

In the next chapter, we'll explore more about what yoga therapy is, and how it can help with PMADs.

CONCLUSION

Reading through this chapter may have been tough. It's painful to acknowledge our suffering, and it takes courage to say, "I have a problem and I need help." Yoga teaches us, however, that bringing light to our darkest places is always wise. Acknowledging our struggles allows us to access the support and treatments that are available. The very good news is that these treatments work, and moms do recover from PMADs—feeling more hope, more joy, more ease, more humor, and more connection to their babies and themselves. Moms who felt disconnected from their babies develop loving, close relationships. Every day as a parent, you develop new skills and new strength to keep going.

Yoga Therapy: A Compassionate Mind-Body Response

If you've picked up this book, you have likely been suffering, dealing with painful and challenging thoughts and feelings. You've turned to this book because you are trying to do something to feel better. You want this time period to be the magical time of love and bonding that you expected. You want to be a good mom. You want your kid to be okay, to feel loved by you, to grow up healthy and securely attached. Of course you want to fix this!

Yoga and mindfulness are often marketed like everything else in commercials, from detergent to milk to self-help books—as something to make us and our children calmer, happier, more efficient, more organized, more successful, more beautiful, skinnier, and in all ways better. The marketing of yoga, in this way, implies that we are not already good enough. Worse, it implies that if we are suffering, we just aren't doing enough yoga.

I'm not going to promise you that yoga will fix you, make you a perfect mom, or prevent you or your child from ever suffering. I'm not going to promise you that you will feel better today, tomorrow, or even any time this week. Yoga and motherhood are mirrors for each other here—if we expect all sunshine and roses, we are in for disappointment. But while the news that there's no quick fix might be a disappointment, we shouldn't be disappointed.

Because openness, compassion, and spaciousness in the face of suffering is even more powerful. The new way of responding—what yoga truly offers—is about softening, not solving.

Think of yoga practice as time spent with a best friend. She sits with you in your sorrow, anger, laughter, tears, mistakes, and triumphs. She doesn't fix anything, but she makes life feel fuller, saner, richer, sweeter. If you are happy, it's a joy to celebrate together. If you are sad, she comforts you. Yoga, your friend, helps you endure. She helps you find moments of beauty and ease in the middle of the muck so that when you look back, you remember some good things about this time.

Yoga is a reward in and of itself.

WHAT IS YOGA?

Poses, or *asanas*, are only the most visible part of yoga practice, which is why they grace the cover of yoga books and magazines. Many modern yoga classes focus entirely on this one part of yoga. But yoga encompasses so much more than poses: it is a set of philosophies and a practical system aimed at awakening consciousness. Yoga is a practice of getting free of misconceptions we have about who we are and how we are supposed to live. We tend to mistake ourselves for being just our bodies, our thoughts, and our achievements. Yoga teaches us that we are all of these things and so much more. We learn to see ourselves as a drop of water in a great ocean, connected to ourselves and to all of humanity.

The word *yoga* actually means "to yoke" or "bring together." We practice inviting our bodies, hearts, and minds to work together toward simple aims, like sitting in meditation or balancing in tree pose, with the grander aim of experiencing and creating clarity, freedom, transcendent spaciousness, and freedom.

Some of the key tools in yoga that you will find in this book are:

- Breathing techniques (*pranayama*)
- Physical movement and body postures (*asana*)
- Inward focus (*pratyahara*) and self-study (*svadyaya*)
- Meditation (*dharana, dhyana*)
- Cultivation of qualities like compassion, truthfulness, and acceptance

It's likely that some of these tools will sound better to you than others. Yoga has been handed down through many lineages, schools, and traditions, each with a path that appeals to different people, with different temperaments and tendencies. For some people, *hatha yoga*, which involves the physical poses and breathwork, is the most accessible. Others might practice *bhakti yoga*, the yoga of singing and devotion; *karma yoga*, the yoga of service; or *jnana yoga*, which involves studying texts. There is no wrong path, and there are many right paths. Much like parenting!

WHAT IS YOGA THERAPY?

Yoga therapy is the application of yoga to support health and healing. Yoga therapy has been shown to be effective for conditions ranging from those thought to be physical, such as back pain or heart problems, to those thought to be emotional, such as depression or anxiety. Because yoga views and treats the person as a whole, someone may come to yoga therapy to heal back pain and find that they feel more at peace in their day-to-day lives. In some cases, yoga cannot "heal" an injury or illness, but can, instead, help practitioners change their relationship to their conditions, finding more ease and freedom as they navigate their care.

Yoga therapists work in many fields of medicine and wellness. They are not just health professionals who practice yoga and apply it in their work—they have specialized training and supervision in how to do so in an effective and ethical manner. Most yoga therapists already have degrees or licenses in their area of practice or expertise and may integrate yoga therapy into other disciplines.

I specialize in using yoga therapy for conditions that are supported by my training as a psychotherapist—PMADs, general stress, depression, anxiety, eating disorders, addiction, and trauma. Yoga therapy can be especially useful for people whose problems have led to a disconnect or even an animosity between mind and body.

In yoga therapy, you practice finding balance and flexibility, both physically and mentally. Through experimentation with and exposure to physical challenge, presence, and stillness, you develop steadiness and resilience in the face of anxiety, self-criticism, and overwhelm. You come to see how your mind works—what patterns, attachments, and aversions are automatic and what might better serve you. You learn to accept and meet your body and mind as they are while simultaneously challenging yourself to grow, change, and build strength. If you have a history of trauma, you slowly recover a sense of agency, choice, integration, and safety in your body. Yoga therapy also invites relaxation, enjoyment in body sensations, and a sense of inner peace. You develop tools that can be used for emotional regulation, self-soothing, and self-knowledge.

Most importantly, yoga therapy supports you in developing your own yoga practice, one that does not depend on or belong to the therapist or therapy room. You hold the power for your own care, healing, and growth. You walk away with therapeutic tools that are now free and portable, and require nothing but themselves.

In reading this book, you will see that much of my approach as a yoga therapist comes from my training in psychology. A student of psychology will surely recognize a lot of existential-humanistic therapy, cognitive behavioral therapy (CBT), mindfulness-based cognitive therapy (MBCT), dialectical behavioral therapy (DBT), and acceptance and commitment therapy (ACT). The latter three of these modern therapy approaches are based in large part on Buddhist mindfulness practice, and so you will notice the influence of mindfulness in the practices offered here as well. I find it endlessly reassuring and fascinating how all these approaches, at their core, suggest similar paths to healing, just using different words.

How Yoga Therapy Can Help

A comprehensive yoga practice can be a powerful framework for healing PMADs because it offers ways to address all the aspects of body, mind, and soul. Yoga offers self-knowledge, behavior change, and biochemical antidepressant effects. If we think about the word *depression*, it comes from the root *press*, meaning to push down, make compact, reduce space. In Sanskrit, similarly, the word *dukha*, or suffering, literally means "obstructed space."[6] Yoga does the opposite of depressing or obstructing space—it uplifts, creates space, and moves against inertia.

Yoga offers these specific tools to a new mama experiencing challenging thoughts and feelings:

- A practice that can hold all struggles without having to push them away: instead of positive thinking, or trying to just be happy, yoga practice is an invitation to all that is present. When we come to practice, sadness is welcome, agitation is welcome. Yoga is inclusionary versus exclusionary. It is a tuning in to our experience, rather than a tuning out.
- Practical self-care for aches and pains (which affect mood)
- Self-compassion
- Exercise, which helps with anxiety and depression
- Relaxation and energizing: when we balance our use of active and passive poses with our moods, we slowly adjust our nervous system so that we feel both of these things at the same time—we are alert but relaxed.
- Valuable insight into self, needs, and moods
- Steadiness in the storm

One hallmark of depression and anxiety is that thoughts feel very real, and we can begin to see our negative worldview as wholly true. We might struggle to imagine seeing things otherwise. Yoga gives us the opportunity to come into touch with the true self, beyond thoughts or worldviews, capable of holding all.

Yogic practices exactly parallel what psychology calls "emotional regulation"—learning to notice and understand how your mind, body, and emotions work, then choosing to adjust yourself in ways that cultivate peace.

It's not all sunshine and rainbows along the way. There is a reason yoga practitioners talk about developing *tapas*, or fire, to maintain a dedicated practice. You can go in expecting all bliss, but the fire will burn at times. You will come face to face with your deepest pain, and still you stay steady on your path, like the hero of your own fairy tale. You may be thinking, *I don't want to face my deepest pain. And I don't have the energy for a dedicated practice.* But before you put this book down, consider that yoga and mothering are alike in that they are both challenging and extremely rewarding. In both arenas, it's when we face our deepest challenges that the magic comes in.

Yoga enhances motherhood and motherhood enhances yoga. Yoga helps heal depression and anxiety, and walking a path of awareness from depression and anxiety toward health enhances yoga. All three—motherhood, healing, and yoga—work as wonderful metaphors, friends, and catalysts for each other.

SOME THOUGHTS ABOUT BALANCING ACCEPTANCE AND CHANGE

During my time as a pregnant and new mom, yoga did help me feel better, calmer, more hopeful, (slightly) more sane, and spiritually connected. It enabled me to be more present and connected to my baby, my husband, and my community. Yet yoga only helped because it welcomed me in my distress. Yoga taught me to stop seeing my messy feelings and thoughts, or my level of calm, as permanent, as my true self, or as signs that I was worthy or unworthy as a person or a parent.

This is the acceptance and change paradox that is at the heart of yoga therapy. Yoga therapy accepts us just as we are, yet offers us a path of change. When I meet as a therapist with new moms, I work hard to provide a space that is fully accepting of them wherever they are, that invites them to share their most difficult feelings. I want them to know that pain and sorrow are necessary parts of being alive. And then I also work on tangible behaviors with them, helping them develop practices that make being alive a little bit easier.

The tension between acceptance and change can also be described as balancing ease and effort. There is a yoga aphorism about this from the *Yoga Sutras of Patanjali,* Sutra 2.46: "*Stirah sukham asanam.*"[7] *Asana,* as you might remember, means pose, posture, or even seat. *Stirah* refers to effort, steadiness, dedication. *Sukham* means ease, sweetness, comfort. So we are told in this sutra to practice both effort and ease in each pose. Because poses serve as metaphors, we can take this to mean that we are encouraged to balance effort and ease in our lives. I've heard many yogis describe *stirah* and *sukham* as two wings of a bird. You need them both to fly.

How apt for surviving the early days of mothering. Some days we must allow ourselves to just let go, stay home, not worry about showering, cleaning the house, exercising, or doing anything tough. Other days, we need to push ourselves to take that shower, to get dressed, to go out, to get our bodies moving. Some days, we need to remind ourselves that we don't have to be perfect mothers, that our babies will be okay if they cry for a few minutes, that our families can cope without us if we take some time just for ourselves to take a nap or go to a yoga class. Other days, we need to talk ourselves into showing up for our family, doing what feels hard, cheerleading ourselves into changing a diaper, feeding the baby, connecting with our loved ones.

I'm hoping this book offers lots of both acceptance and change strategies, and if you find yourself getting stuck on one, start by noticing that. If I'm talking about how you can invite in a difficult feeling, you may note that you think, *No way! I need these feelings to go away!* If I'm talking about a way to care for your difficult feeling, you might want to say, "That's not going to work! Stop trying to fix me!" Notice both of these responses, and smile at your humanity. Know that everyone responds that way, and then come back to the moment. If an idea is helpful right now, great. If not, ignore it for now. It's always here if you want to come back to it.

This book challenges you to approach both yoga and motherhood this way: do your absolute best, and at the same time, let go of trying to be good. Focus on "good enough."

HOW TO APPROACH THE PRACTICES IN THIS BOOK

There are more than fifty yoga practices offered in this book. You might feel overwhelmed by that. Where should you start?

Take What You Like

As you read through the book, take note of which practices appeal to you, or seem like they might be useful or doable. Pick up a few practices here and there to use as coping skills. Try them out and find which ones might work for you in the moment. If you like, dog-ear the page or write them on a Post-it note. Use them whenever you need them. Even if you don't try them for weeks and weeks, they are always there, available to you. Maybe they work. Maybe they don't. Don't feel any pressure to keep using a tool that doesn't feel right to you. Yoga has something for everybody.

For some readers, especially those who aren't that "into" yoga, reading the first part of each chapter and taking in the validation of parenting struggles will actually be all that you need. Self-compassion and self-understanding can be very healing even if you don't read or try any of the practices in each chapter.

Be Safe

Listen to what feels safe for your body. Pick something that is appropriate for where you are in your pregnancy or postpartum state. I tried to focus as much as possible on practices that were accessible at most stages of the pregnancy and postpartum period, but I did include and note some that you just couldn't do comfortably at all stages or in every body. Skip those and come back to them when it is more appropriate. There are so many options here, including those that don't require you to use your body at all. Be mindful of injuries and reach out to a competent yoga teacher if you need more guidance. You may want to check in with your care providers for advice as well.

Experiment

When you pick up a book about yoga therapy, you might expect there to be a list of specific poses you should use for different issues to fix them. For example, *if you are sad, do a warrior II; if you are tired, do a headstand.*

This book has some of that, but not much. That's too prescriptive. That's like a dream interpretation book saying that every dream about teeth falling out is about control. Every pose feels really different for every body. People work different ways, have different life experiences and patterns that affect how we respond to a pose. An inversion might be calming for one person and bring fear and anxiety to another. Yoga therapy should always be an individualized process.

When you try one of the practices offered, trust that you will respond in your own (sometimes unexpected) way, and view this as a general process of trial and error. You may even find that a pose helps you in a way that is totally different from its "intended purpose." After all, each practice could help with multiple things—that warrior II might be great if you are sad *and* great if you are anxious. It could also help with your tight pregnant hips. I've often heard it said in yoga therapy circles that yoga doesn't have side effects—it has side benefits.

Keep It Simple

One of the biggest roadblocks to starting yoga or any contemplative practice is getting past how these practices are marketed. We see images of skinny, flexible, white acrobats doing poses on the beach at sunset and think, *No way. That's not me.*

Change your idea of what yoga should look like. Do not set a goal of "doing yoga" like you do in a yoga class. Don't set the expectation that "real" yoga takes ninety minutes a day. (That timing is just what works for studios.) A "deeper" or "more advanced" practice is not one that takes longer, occurs in a studio, or involves having open hamstrings. A deep practice is one that you can actually maintain and do often.

It will be easier to have a regular yoga practice if your goals are modest. One minute of meditation every day is much better than expecting an hour and beating yourself up when you don't do it.

Choose a few (and when I say a few, I mean about three) practices from this book, and put them together into a committed, steady home practice. Only add more if you start to yearn for more, and be willing to let "more" go on a difficult day.

Don't change it up too often. One of the most important parts of yoga therapy is responding to your needs and being willing to change. But once you've settled on a practice that suits you, resist urges to commit to something else, at least for a few weeks. You can go crazy trying to pick the "perfect" practice, because there is no such thing. Especially when you have anxiety, making choices can be difficult and the need to make it "just right" can be paralyzing. Let the ones you've committed to be good enough.

If you really can't decide, I'll choose for you. Here is a balanced home yoga practice that you can start with:

- One minute of basic can't-fail meditation (page 71)
- One minute of belly breathing (page 75)
- Five rounds of cat/cow (page 165)

Reserve Your Time

When I describe yoga practices, I rarely tell you how long to practice them. This is because everyone's needs vary. Most of these practices can be useful when practiced any length, from one breath to one hour. The worst distraction when practicing, however, is constantly looking at the clock. I suggest you set a timer for the amount of time you'd like to practice. Then, trust the timer, and do your best not to look at it repeatedly to see how much time you have left. This will prevent you from giving up too soon or forcing yourself to go much longer than you need to. Setting a timer will help you to build confidence and let go of striving.

Another way to set the time of your practice is to do it while something happens. For example, choose a time limit like "I'll do this pose for five breaths," "I'll do this breath practice until my baby finishes this bottle," "I'll practice till my baby wakes up" or "Every time I pee, I'll take three belly breaths before leaving the bathroom."

Some people find that it also helps to set a time of day to practice, like the first five minutes when they wake up in the morning, or the last five before bed. Other ideas I've heard are: during a baby's nap, while nursing, for three minutes in your car before you get out of it, before dinner, or for ten minutes before you watch TV.

Whet Your Appetite

I once heard that we should replace the English word *discipline* as it relates to yoga with the word *appetite*. Instead of searching for the discipline to practice, we can search for the appetite to practice. The dictionary definition of discipline—"training to develop a skill"—can be a useful way to think about practice. We do yoga to develop skills—of returning to the present moment, of being able to discern what is right for us and our children, of connecting better to others with less drama and more empathy. These are all lovely ways to think about discipline. For most of us, however, the word *discipline* tends to bring up more of a sense of forcing ourselves to do something because we must improve. We think, *I should do yoga. Because I'm bad if I don't. Because I'm only good—actually, only okay—if I do.*

Appetite, on the other hand, implies that the desire to practice comes from a place within. That our bodies and hearts yearn to be nourished by a practice. Just as an appetite for food, when truly listened to, will tell us when we are satisfied, when is enough, so an appetite for yoga will tell us just what our bodies and minds need, without focus on achievement.

Look for practices that make your mind think, *Ah, that would be great.* Even if you have to work sometimes to bring yourself to practice or to stay with the practice, does it feel like it gives you something back? A sense of spaciousness, release, ease, strength, compassion, or connection to yourself or others?

Use the Word *Practice*

Using the word *practice* reminds us we cannot turn yoga into just one more thing we are not doing perfectly enough. Saying we practice gives us permission to be playful, to experiment, to try again. We get very clear with ourselves that this is not ever about being good at yoga or meditation—it's just about, well, practicing. We make time and space to practice and that's enough.

Find satisfaction in the here and now in your practice, rather than only looking to the improvement or the outcome. Perhaps seek to emulate your baby—hungering to master new tasks: grasping a toy, putting spoon to mouth, eagerly taking first steps, falling and yet delighting in the journey. When was the last time you heard a three-month-old baby insisting, "I've failed! I should be able to walk by now!"

Keep It Up!

I don't want anyone reading this to feel like they aren't doing this right if they only use these tools every once in awhile. However, I always feel sad when someone tries a yoga tool once or twice, still feels anxious or depressed, and then dismisses it, saying "It didn't work," and giving up on yoga. Though many of these tools will "work" when used on occasion to end a panic attack or lift you out of a particularly bad mood, many of them are like medications that have to build up in your system to achieve maximum effect.

Practicing yoga regularly, with dedication, brings a deeper transformation over time. A consistent practice, or *sadhana,* shows you that yoga can hold anything—because you practice on sad days and happy days, it builds your patience, your endurance, your resilience, and your flexibility. It makes the practices seem like second nature, so that when you need them to "work," they are easy to remember and grasp. Just like our relationships with our new babies, yoga unfolds over time, revealing new layers each time we practice.

If you enthusiastically start a practice, and then a week or two later lose momentum and stop, please forgive yourself. Know that you can come back to the practice any time.

Remind yourself to think of yoga practice as a friendship. The more regular time you spend with your friend, tending to the friendship, the deeper your connection grows. Sometimes you don't keep up with a friend. You get busy, you don't return a phone call, and then you feel worried that you can't reach out again, that maybe the friend is mad at you or the connection is gone. But likely, if you just reach out again, you and your friend, just like you and your yoga practice, can begin again. Maybe the spark of connection comes back right away, or maybe it takes some time to warm up and feel comfortable again.

Go for the Combo

Practicing the things in this book does not mean you need to stop your therapy or medications. One thing will complement and strengthen the other. Get all the help you need—from your community and from professionals. There are no medals for doing this alone.

CONCLUSION

I hope that, after reading this, you have a new idea about yoga—that it sounds like something you could actually begin experimenting with right now, today. If you still notice yourself thinking that you have to go to a ninety-minute class, or that you should have started this sooner, or that this is something that only helps happy, fit, flexible people whose laundry is already done, please know you are in good company. It's hard for so many of us to let go of old concepts and to be vulnerable enough to hope. Remind yourself that yoga is not here to demand things of you, judge you, or fix you. Yoga is here to be a supportive companion, a source of soothing and strength, a well of sanity. Yoga therapy is here for you, right now, just as you are. All you have to do is begin.

part two
The Practices

Section One
Make a Plan for Practice and for Support

The first step for any mom in healing from PMADs is to get support—
from professionals, friends, family, community, and, possibly, a yoga
practice. Because life with a new baby can be hectic and overwhelming,
it helps a lot to take time out to set up a plan to make sure that you have
that support available. In section 1, you will learn how to set up a simple
yoga practice that will support you. We will explore how to meditate, how
to do basic breathwork, how yoga poses can work to help you transform
difficult experiences, and how to integrate these practices into this time
of intensively mothering your baby.

Where do I begin?

The way to begin healing from anxiety and depression is just like the way to begin a yoga practice: start now. Don't wait until things get worse. Don't wait until things get better. Don't put it off till you feel like it, till you are getting more sleep, till you are in "better shape," till it doesn't feel scary. If you wait until you are "ready" for it, you will be waiting forever.

Begin today, in your imperfect state, as you are.

Yoga therapy starts with raising awareness of what is going on with you. Are you experiencing depression, fatigue, exhaustion, inertia? Or are you feeling anxious, irritable, turbulent, wound-up, worried? Or a combination of both? Or different feelings at different times of day or in different circumstances?

Let your state guide you into your first practice. Because PMADs can take many forms, there is no one "good practice" for healing. There are, however, two good paths to take in choosing how to start: (1) meeting yourself where you are, and (2) taking opposite action.

"Meeting yourself where you are" is a path that works when resistance is high. If the idea of doing yoga (or anything else) sounds exhausting, overwhelming, or perhaps impossible, start with things that are gentle and slow. Find practices in this book you can do without moving or without getting out of bed. Let the practices you choose be a soft embrace of yourself as you are. If you feel anxious, and stopping your busyness seems scary, find practices that feel productive, such as combining exercise with mindfulness, or meditations you can do while you move through your life.

"Taking opposite action" is a tool that comes from dialectical behavior therapy, or DBT[8], a form of psychotherapy. Opposite action maps onto one of the most basic principles of yoga therapy—that like increases like and opposites bring balance.

Maybe depression gives you an urge to avoid people or stay in your PJs all day. Maybe rage gives you an urge to yell at people. Maybe anxiety gives you an urge to be constantly busy, never stopping or slowing down. Many of us believe that to change these urges, we have to change the feeling behind them. We wait (and wait and wait) until we don't feel depressed anymore to get out and about. We wait until we don't feel anxious to sit down and rest. Opposite action tells us that, actually, you can change your behavior without changing your feelings first. Sometimes, changing behavior *now* changes your feelings later.

If you'd like to try opposite action, you'd choose a practice that you might have to push yourself a little bit to do. It might sound intimidating or tiring, but something in it seems like it might shake you out of a stuck place. Maybe you choose a meditation practice even though sitting still sounds hard, or you do a vigorous movement practice even though you are tired. You apply what in yoga is called *tapas*, an effortful oomph to help you along.

Neither of these paths is right, and neither is wrong. They are just two options. Yoga has always offered many paths to healing and liberation. You can choose one path, and then later choose another. The important thing is to begin.

Practice Choose a Path

Sit with yourself in quiet, perhaps closing your eyes or taking a soft gaze at the floor.

Ask yourself:

What am I feeling?

What is my suffering like?

What do I feel might help me?

What do I feel capable of?

What is the most loving gesture for myself today: meeting myself where I am, or taking opposite action?

What would give me a sense of hope?

Keep your answers in mind as you read the practices in this book, helping you choose which tools and ideas you would like to try on.

You don't need a reason, and it's not your fault

One of the most common refrains I hear from moms when they are suffering from depression or anxiety is, "I have no reason to be depressed. I have everything I've ever wanted. I have this beautiful baby. I should be grateful." Then, because no reason has been uncovered, "This is my fault—something is wrong with me." The "wrong with me" most moms come up with is that they are selfish, unloving, ungrateful, bad mothers.

But really—you do not need to have a reason to be anxious or depressed. No one asks to have depression or anxiety. It's not your fault. I've heard it said that you don't choose PMADs, they choose you.

Searching for a reason can become just another way to leave the present moment, to bargain ourselves out of reality. We can get caught up in *I'll be happy when* or *I'd be happy if I hadn't* thoughts—*I'd be happy if we hadn't moved here, I'll be happy when my house is clean, I'll be happy when the baby sleeps through the night, I'll be happy at the end of my work week, I'll be happy when the sitter gets here.*

Yoga teaches us to accept that suffering is part of life—not because you are flawed in a way someone else isn't, but because your brain, like all human brains, tends to do things like compare, strive, stick. You also have a human body, vulnerable to injury and illness. When suffering is up big time, no matter why, we can greet ourselves in the present moment as we are. We can tend to ourselves and offer compassion.

Yoga asks us to detach our problems from ourselves—to see them not as who we are, but rather as conditions, stuck patterns of thinking or behaving. Our problems are like a veil that makes it hard to see everything in reality clearly. We don't notice a veil in front of us because we can look right through it. Yoga teaches us to notice the veil—to observe how we work. This practice, called *svadhyaya*, or self-study, is at the heart of the yoga therapy approach.

When we can let go of blaming ourselves for having depression or anxiety, or for suffering, when we can let go of trying to figure out and fix what might have happened to get us here, when we can stop wondering if we deserve to get support and help, then we can face the truth of what is happening, and address it. We can ask, "What do I need to survive this? What do I need to access my true self?" We can focus on getting the help and care that we need.

Practice **Quick Body-Mind-Heart Self-Study**

I offer this meditation at the beginning of every yoga class I teach, and share it with all of my therapy clients. It can be done any time, any place, and quickly (though it can be nice to sink in to it, when you have more time). It can serve you when you are calm or when feelings are strong. Doing it many times a day helps keep you in touch with yourself and what you might need.

Close your eyes or take a soft gaze at the floor.

Body Notice what is happening in your body. Don't try to change anything, just notice. Where do you feel tension or relaxation? What is your energy level? What temperature are you?

Mind Notice thoughts in your mind: stories, themes, words, and images. No need to label them as good or bad, rational or irrational, just notice.

Heart What emotions do you have? Can you label the emotion in one or two words (like anger or joy)? How strong is the emotion? Where do you feel it in your body? Let go of judgment. Welcome whatever is there with your awareness.

Now, broaden your awareness to take in all of what is happening right now—body, mind, heart, breath, perhaps baby in your belly or your arms. Breathe here as long as you like, with spacious awareness, watching sensations, thoughts, and emotions come and go.

Practice **Mindful Journaling**

You can connect with your observing mind by writing out what you notice in your body, mind, and heart. Writing can make the concept of observer more concrete, easier to identify. Here is an example of mindful journaling—something I wrote when my daughter was ten months old and had kept me up much of the night as a new tooth emerged:

I am so tired—my brain in a bit of a fog as I sit to write. It takes me twice as long as it usually would to form sentences. I notice a deep ache of desire for sleep. Sticky, rapid thoughts of resentment—at my partner, at my older daughter, at myself for not figuring out this sleep situation earlier. I notice a sadness and yearning for more than this precious hour for myself, and a jealousy of those who have more time. I notice my shoulders feel tight and achy from holding, my nipples a bit tender from nursing. I notice that I have a faint smell of milk, and that the recognition of this smell brings a smile to my face, a sweet wish to be holding my baby again, and sense of what the weight of her soft head in my arms would be, the texture of her fine, short hair on the skin of my palms. I notice that I am fantasizing both about seeing her soon and about having the rest of the day to myself to do whatever I want.

No, you won't "just be fine"

In preparation for labor, many moms make a "birth plan," a hopeful list of preferences for what they'd like to do and how they'd like to be treated in labor. The idea is that during labor, they may not be able to speak up and advocate for themselves, so they can ask their partners and providers to look to the plan for guidance.

Birth lasts for a maximum of, say, three days. The postnatal period, however, is much longer—yet no one writes down a plan for that! Most moms just say, "I'll be fine. I don't need to plan." PMADs, however, bring inertia, brain fog, and overwhelm; babies take up all your time; and having a plan may mean the difference between caring for yourself and not. As with a birth plan, share this with partners and providers in case you are not able to put it in place yourself. This plan can include things that are nourishing and preventative, as well as what to do if you are suffering.

Even if you didn't plan ahead and you pick this book up when you have an eight-month-old, it's never too late to make a plan. Sit down with your partner or support folks and write down how you will care for yourself, social and professional resources you can access, what your yoga/meditation practice will be, and what help you will need to stick with it.

SAMPLE PMADs PLAN

Social support (write down at least two friends or family members in each category, and show them this plan):

- Friends to set up meal support, using an online "Meal Train" or a phone tree

- Friends who can visit and hold the baby while I nap or shower, do laundry, straighten the house
- Friends who I want to know I am struggling, who I need to come to rally around me; I'm okay with my partner or family calling these friends and telling them what's going on if I am not able to.
- I will check in every night with my partner or support person to talk about how we are feeling and what kind of help we each need, and to offer appreciations.

Family and friends can remind me:

- You are doing a great job
- You are good enough
- I love you
- It's okay to get help

Professional support (write down one or two names in each category):

- Therapist specializing in helping new parents (LCSW, MFT, PsyD, PhD)
- Psychiatrist who specializes in reproductive medicine, or an obstetrician with significant mental health knowledge. Talk to potential providers and find out how up to date they are on reproductive mental health.
- Holistic health: chiropractor, massage therapist, acupuncturist or low-fee community acupuncture clinic, sleep consultant, lactation consultant
- Postpartum doula or night nurse
- Childcare
- PMADs support group
- Hotline/warmline number I can call: Postpartum Support International 1-800-944-4773(4PPD)

Family balance:

- Even in this day and age, and even when both parents work, mothers are often left with a greater amount of the cooking, housework, bill paying, care for older children, and remembering doctor appointments, family birthdays, and the like. I can challenge these automatic roles. Here is my plan for how to work toward sharing these tasks equitably with my partner, or how to get outside help. I may also need someone to take on an extra share of these duties while I heal.

  - Cooking/groceries:
  - Cleaning:
  - Laundry:
  - Scheduling appointments:
  - Setting up childcare:
  - Paying bills:
  - Other:

Helpful activities:

- Showering daily
- Sleep—work out a plan to get at least eight hours over the course of twenty-four
- Home yoga practice
- Postpartum or Mom & Baby yoga class (find out when and where it meets, how to sign up)
- New moms group or meet-up
- Gym/exercise studio with childcare (many YMCAs offer this)
- Baby classes: music, massage, Gymboree, storytime, etc.

Supplies:

- At least two good water bottles that do not require using hands to drink from
- Lots of pillows, so that my back and elbows are always supported when feeding or holding my baby
- Frozen food and easy snacks, so I never have to be hungry
- Nice music to have on in the background during the day
- Slip-on shoes

Practice **Yoga Plan**

For any yoga practitioner, committing to a practice plan is essential to maintaining a home practice in their busy lives—this is doubly true when you have a baby. This book contains so many possible practices that you may struggle to choose. Write down a plan to do a few and let go of the rest of them. Here is an example of a plan:

Home practice
I commit to three yoga practices a day. These can be short, and I am not allowed to bully myself into doing them. They are breaks that are just for me. (Note: all practices below can be found elsewhere in the book. Page numbers are noted in parentheses.)

One meditation or mindfulness practice, like
- Quick body-mind-heart self-study (page 63)
- "Focus on the light within" meditation (page 89)
- Feeding meditation (page 220)

One breathing practice, like
- Breath cycle awareness (page 82)
- Belly breathing (page 75)

- Bee breath (page 204)
- Alternate nostril breathing (page 205)

One movement practice, like
- Sun salutations (page 223)
- Simple mindful movements (page 104)
- Warrior II (page 79)
- Keep-ups (page 117)
- Downward-facing dog (page 223)
- Restorative child's pose (page 200)

Sample sequences:

Pregnant
"Focus on the light within" meditation

Belly breathing

Keep-ups

After birth
Quick body-mind-heart self-study

Breath cycle awareness

Simple mindful movements

With three-month-old
Mindful feeding

Bee breath

Five sun salutations

I can ask for help to make time for this. I have asked someone (partner, friend, family member) to check in with me and see if I need them to care for the baby while I do my practice.

It is easier to practice with a sangha, or community. I could ask my partner or a family member to practice with me every day, turning it into a family ritual.

If and when I'd like a longer practice, I can consult a teacher, use a video, or put together a longer sequence to do at home.

I'm not good at meditation

You have probably been told, maybe many times, that you *should* meditate or try mindfulness. Maybe you took a meditation class once a few years ago and thought everything the teacher said was cheesy and never looked back. Maybe you meditated for years and loved it—but somewhere along the way, you stopped or decided, *I'm not good at it.*

I am going to offer here the simplest, least cheesy form of meditation I know. But first, we need to bust a few myths.

Myth #1 I'm not good at meditation.
Answer There is no such thing as being good at meditating. There are no grades or rewards. This is a practice for you, not an achievement.

Myth #2 My mind just can't be clear.
Answer Great. YOU DO NOT NEED TO HAVE A CLEAR MIND. No one has a clear mind. That would be of great concern and require medical attention. Even people who have meditated for years have troublesome, sticky, annoying thoughts. It's part of the deal of being human.

Myth #3 I don't have time.
Answer First, I definitely want to validate that you have no free time. The good news is that you do not need to have free time to meditate. I'm sure you have one minute that you are spending each day looking at your phone. If you used just that one minute to meditate, that would be good enough. Not just a good start—good enough. One minute a day *is* a meditation practice. You don't have to meditate for a long time or be somewhere special to meditate.

Do not, I repeat do not, tell yourself that you are going to make a nice peaceful corner of your home for meditating, and you will start as soon as you set up your altar and clean all the laundry out of the way. If you have a to-do list for meditating, let go of it. You can meditate sitting on a pile of laundry. You can meditate if a baby is in your arms. You can meditate if a baby is screaming in your arms. You don't need it to be quiet or pretty or calm. Those things are great—how wonderful if you can get some quiet, and beauty, and peace for yourself—but not necessary.

Practice **Basic Can't-Fail Meditation**

Set an alarm for a reasonable period of time. You decide what reasonable is. One minute is fine. Fifteen minutes is fine. Three minutes and twenty-three seconds is fine.

- Sit down. Or lie down. Or get still.
- Close your eyes or pick a spot on the floor to gaze at.
- Notice your breath.
- Now your mind wanders: it may think about your clothes, your dinner, politics, the fight you had with your partner, how tired you are, if you are doing this right, or how much you suck at meditating.
- As soon as you notice this, say to yourself, "Oh, I notice myself thinking. Now I'm going back to my breath."
- Notice your breath.
- Now your mind wanders again.
- Again, as soon as you notice this, say to yourself, "Oh, I notice myself thinking. Now I'm going back to my breath."
- Now your mind wanders again. You may become very annoyed with your mind. That's okay.
- Again, as soon as you notice this, say to yourself, "Oh, I notice myself thinking. Now I'm going back to my breath."

The point of meditation is not to not think; it is to notice that we are thinking. Every time you notice a thought, you are doing what is supposed to happen in the meditation. Imagine you get a point every time you notice that you are thinking. Then maybe you will feel like you are winning when you notice a thought, instead of thinking it means you are failing!

This kind of meditation is good practice for accepting that you do not have to be peaceful or happy all the time to be a good enough mom. When you meditate, it's an act of taking care of yourself that is unconditional—you sit down and meditate and don't judge your goodness by the outcome of a peaceful mind. Just like you take care of your baby and don't judge your goodness by the outcome of a baby that smiles and coos and never cries.

Over time, you learn how your mind works and what patterns come up. You intimately experience how intense feelings swell up and then pass away, rather than just saying, "This too shall pass." You might learn, *Wow, I have this one story that comes up over and over.* Then you can see it as a story and say, "Here it comes again," rather than attaching to it, analyzing it, or trying to push it away.

Unlike in a physical yoga practice, in which beginner poses are often followed by progressively more challenging poses, after a long time meditating, there is no need to move to "harder" practices. The basic act of watching the breath can be enough for a lifetime. More experienced meditators may, instead, develop tolerance and willingness to meditate for longer periods of time. Please don't put pressure on yourself to do that! There are many seasons in life, and the season of the childbearing years is not one in which you need pressure to do more.

If you try meditation many times, and it brings up an intolerable amount of anxiety for you, that's great information. You may decide to stick with it, this time aware that you are applying the principle of opposite action, knowing that over time, a regular meditation practice does quite often help relieve anxiety. Alternately, you may decide this is a great opportunity to practice the principle of meeting your-self where you are at. You might choose instead to do more active, movement-based practices to allow your body to move with the anx-ious energy.

All you have to do is breathe

We all know that in moments of distress, it helps to take a deep breath. This seems obvious. So why are we talking about it?

Because, in the depths of struggle, we often forget that the breath is right there for us, ready to help us find balance, ease, and energy.

It truly amazes me that something so holy, so life-affirming, so profound, is also something we just do all day long, without trying. Breath sustains us, with or without our attention, always available for a moment of transcendence if we look for it. The breath is the one new-mom essential that you don't have to remember to pack in your diaper bag when you leave the house.

In Sanskrit, the word for breath is *prana*, which also means life-force. Indeed, breath not only provides a spiritual anchor, but it is also what gives us life. Just as it is a miracle when a baby comes out and takes their first breath, so it is a miracle every time you take a breath and find yourself alive.

Breathing practices in yoga are called *pranayama*. *Yama* means restraint or regulation. *Pranayama* is the regulation of the breath and life-force. Regulating our life-force can consciously shift our experience in the moment, like a thermostat for your nervous system. Slow breathing calms you. Breathing faster revs you up.

My "aha" moments with yoga in pregnancy and postpartum don't have much to do with poses. They all have to do with the breath. In the depths of my pregnancy nausea, in the storm of labor contractions, in the monotony of early breastfeeding, when I was just about to leave the house and my baby pooped all over me, when my toddler was throwing a loud temper tantrum just as my newborn was falling asleep—an awareness and connection to just one breath provided a moment of space and a sense that I could survive. Breath offers me a break, a world that is all mine, a sense of relief, of drinking in solace, even a taste of delight.

Practice Noticing the Natural Rhythm of Your Breath

No need to start breath practice with special breathing. Just observe your regular breath with a sense of curiosity, as though this is the first breath you've ever taken.

Notice: what happens in the body as you breathe in? Notice your nostrils, chest, ribs, belly, and pelvic floor. How does the body make space to accommodate new air? If you are pregnant, notice specifically how the body in its current form makes space—as the baby fills your belly, where does the air go?

Notice: what happens as you breathe out? How does the body contract to expel old air?

Notice rhythm. Is the inhale longer? The exhale? Are they the same?

Notice how the breath makes you feel.

Practice Belly Breathing

We are born knowing how to belly breathe. Watch your baby—it's just how they breathe! Babies' bellies rise as they inhale, and fall as they exhale. We learn to breathe shallowly some time in childhood, when we are told to hold in our bellies. Shallow breathing only lets us breathe into our chest, simulating a gasp—it tells our bodies that we are not safe to relax. Belly breathing fills up our entire lungs and lets our body know that we have time and space to slow down, and the nervous system often follows by becoming more relaxed. It's as close to a "quick fix" for stress as we can get. Because belly breathing also engages the abdominal muscles, it happens to be a great practice for core strength in the prenatal and postnatal period.

- As you inhale, allow the breath to fill the lungs and expand your belly.
- As you exhale, invite your belly button in to slowly let the air out of the body

If you find yourself doing the opposite, go easy on yourself—many people have forgotten how to purposefully belly breathe. Try putting your hands on your abdomen with the middle fingers on either side of your belly button, about a dime's distance apart. As you inhale, feel the belly expand so that your middle fingers are now a quarter's distance apart. As you exhale, draw the belly muscles in until your middle fingers touch.

Lying down is the easiest position to try this. (In fact, it is hard not to belly breathe lying down.) After you get used to it lying down, you can try practicing it sitting upright. Over time, you can play with belly breathing in all different yoga postures and life circumstances until it becomes second nature.

For some of us, focusing on the breath or taking deep breaths can feel overstimulating or anxiety-provoking. If this is you, take this great opportunity for self-study, to choose other practices, to figure out and respond to what your unique body and mind need.

Affirmations are annoying

Affirmations can be annoying! I notice that any affirmation always makes me want to say the opposite of the affirmation. If someone asks me to say, "I can do it!" I want to say, "But what if I can't?" If I say, "I am peaceful," I feel agitated. And "I am filled with gratitude" just fills me up with complaints.

Many people with depression or anxiety feel this way. In fact, research has shown that when people with low self-esteem say affirmations, they feel worse! They feel invalidated and then get angry at themselves for not being more positive.[9] If you also find affirmations annoying or too theoretical, you can rest assured that you don't have to force yourself to feel "filled with abundance."

None of this is to say that we don't have the ability to bring about a more positive state for ourselves. Perhaps my favorite thing about yoga poses is their infinite ability to provide metaphors that help us work through our struggles tangibly, in an embodied way. The mat becomes a playground, a mirror, and a microcosm. Engaging in specific practices puts us right up against our attachments and aversions, our fears and insecurities. It gives us a safe space to experiment with new ways of being. We can try on the feelings that we want to have. If we want to feel strong, we can use a yoga pose to literally connect to our strength and perseverance. If we want to feel more open and expansive, we can choose a pose in which our limbs reach outward and our chest curves open and up.

Practice **Choose an Asana Metaphor**

Get creative! Choose a pose or movement practice to help develop a quality you need. If you don't have a lot of familiarity with poses to use, this book will give you a lot of options. You can also learn poses from public classes, Here are some ideas:

Strength Try a warrior II (described below) or a plank pose (page 224), or something that accesses your power. Experience viscerally that you can handle challenges.

Patience Choose a challenging pose and practice gradual "mastery" (page 229), watching your progress slowly unfold.

Flexibility Choose an area of your body that feels stuck or tight. Find a pose that stretches it. See how it opens up a little bit more each day.

Responsiveness In a public class, use lots of props and take child's pose (page 200) whenever your body asks for it.

Comparison Do what your mind tells you is the "easiest" version of every pose. Notice thoughts that come up and hold back from physically competing with others (or yourself).

Balance Practice a balance pose. Notice what you do when you fall and how you find your center.

Shift in perspective Do an inversion. How does the world look different from upside down?

Letting go Literally put your feet up in a resting posture, such as legs up the wall (page 201).

Relaxation Go through any set of poses, noticing what happens with your shoulders. Maybe the way you notice that your shoulders hike up in warrior pose primes you to notice how you hike your shoulders up when your kid spills food on the floor for the tenth time today. And you get one second faster at releasing them.

Ability to overcome inertia Lie down in savasana, final resting pose (page 128). Sink into it. You may have the idea that you'll never get up, but it may not be true. See what happens—do you lie there forever? Or, get yourself moving, face the fear of exhaustion, and do five sun salutations (page 223).

Practice **Warrior II**

My favorite pose when I need to feel open or strong is warrior II. I love the sense of being centered while my limbs pull in each direction, arms shooting out like rays of light from my heart. I love the grounding of the feet while the spine reaches tall. I love how the gaze right out over the middle finger feels sharp, focused, and clear.

I often share warrior II with my clients because it works at all stages of pregnancy, and can easily be done with a baby in a carrier. I've even seen students in my Mom & Baby yoga class breastfeed while doing it.

I once had a client who felt that she wasn't as on top of her job as she used to be before motherhood. Since taking maternity leave, she had difficulty speaking up or sharing her opinions with her boss. After doing a warrior pose in our therapy session, she commented that she wished she felt as strong at work as she did in warrior pose. She got the idea to do a warrior pose in her office every morning before she went to talk to her boss. This helped her rediscover her professional identity.

Another postpartum client said she felt gross, tired, weak, and bloated. She felt a lot of disgust toward her new mom body. But when she did a

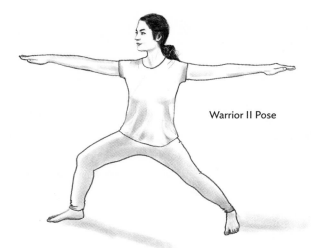

Warrior II Pose

warrior pose, she felt strong and beautiful. Something about starting each day with warrior pose helped her feel together enough to carry on.

To take a warrior pose:
- Begin standing straight on two feet, in what we call mountain pose.
- Step the left foot back about three to four feet. If you feel any discomfort by your pubic bone, you can keep the feet closer together.
- Right toes face forward, and left toes turn slightly out to the left. The left heel is on the floor and the foot stays firmly anchored.
- Bend the right knee forward, no further than your ankle. You might encourage the right thigh to externally rotate, so that the right knee is opening toward the pinkie-toe side of the foot.
- Reach the arms out wide over the legs, perpendicular to the floor, then gaze over the middle finger on the right hand. You may notice a tendency for your torso to follow your gaze, leaning you toward the right fingers. If so, experiment with keeping the torso more upright.

Notice how the pose feels in your body. If this doesn't make you feel strong, what pose does? Maybe something that activates your arms? Play around and take the shape that feels grounding to you.

I never feel good anymore

A cardinal symptom of depression is lack of pleasure when doing things you used to enjoy. Many new moms don't even know if they have this symptom because they no longer have time or energy to do things they used to enjoy. You might miss your old self or believe that you aren't fun anymore. Sexual pleasure might be different, too—you aren't as into it, or what used to feel good feels uncomfortable now. Maybe having your baby nurse or touch you all day leads to feeling "touched out," and you don't even want your partner to attempt to touch you in a way that used to feel good.

Moms who love yoga often tell me they felt it was justifiable to do yoga "for themselves" while pregnant because it was also "for the baby." And they might feel okay going to a mom/baby yoga class. But if they think about going to a regular class *alone*? Guilt. If they do go, the only way to feel okay about it is to take a power yoga class that they can justify as a "workout." Everything has to feel productive.

Make space to do small, unproductive things for yourself that might feel good. Start with your senses. Place things you like to look at, like flowers or art, around your home. Listen to soothing music that you like, instead of baby music. (Your baby won't know the difference!) Wear something soft, cozy, or silky to the touch. Use your favorite shampoo. Savor a piece of chocolate.

Find a way to remind yourself of what makes you happy, of what makes you *you*. Put out pictures of yourself dancing or rock climbing. Set some goals to start up a creative project. Put it on your calendar for two years from now, if you want. If you're worried about neglecting your kids, remind yourself that it is good for them to see you as a full person.

If it's hard to tap into what feels good, your yoga practice can assist you in noticing.

Practice **Breath Cycle Awareness**

The cycle of breath has four parts:

Inhale
Top of the inhale (the pause at the end of the inhale, when you are
full of air)
Exhale
Bottom of the exhale (the pause at the end of the exhale, when you are
empty of air)

I like to imagine the breath as a big Ferris wheel: you ride the cart slowly
up to the top, then back down and around again. You could also think of it as
the moon, waxing and waning.

To practice breath cycle awareness:
- Let your breath fall into its natural rhythm.
- Begin to notice the cycle of breath and what each part feels like.
Inhale, top of the inhale, exhale, bottom of the exhale.
- To amplify awareness, you can experiment with *kumbhaka* or breath
retention. On your next breath, extend the top of the inhale just a bit
longer, holding the air in—then, at the bottom of the exhale, holding the
air out. When you are pregnant, it's best not to do this for very long, just a
second or two, long enough to notice what it feels like.
- As you become more familiar with these four movements of the
breath, you may notice a pattern—that you prefer certain parts of the
breath and don't like others. Maybe the inhale feels nourishing, and
the exhale draining. Maybe the exhale feels relaxing, and the inhale
overwhelming. Retentions might feel scary or peaceful. Maybe you love
that first second of the exhale or the inhale, but don't like it as it goes on.
In my experience, people vary greatly in terms of what part of the breath
they like. It can even shift in one person throughout the day. There is no
right or wrong part to like!

Noticing your preferences with the cycle of breath strengthens your ability to notice what feels good, what you like and don't like. It gives you experiential awareness of the fact that nothing unpleasant lasts forever and that just because something pleasant ends doesn't mean that it isn't coming back. It also gives you practice noticing your attachments without judgment.

You might take this curiosity about your preferences into yoga movement practice. Do a sun salutation (page 223) and notice what parts you like and don't like. Maybe stay in a pose you like for a little longer.

Practice **Juicy Hips**

I learned this one from my wonderful teacher Jane Austin. She teaches "juicy hips" as a way to prevent aching and tightness in the hips and legs and to increase flexibility and range of motion, as well as in preparation for moving through labor. I notice when I teach this movement in my yoga classes, the mamas start smiling and laughing—it's hard not to feel pleasure when your "juices" are flowing!

- Come to hands and knees. You can have your hands on blocks if you like.
- Step one foot forward, outside your hand. The toes can point out slightly.
- Begin to rotate the hips in a circular motion, making the movement as big as you'd like. If you feel any pulling in your pubic area, make the movements much smaller, or point the toes forward.
- Bring your attention to your hips, noticing which part of the circle feels the most "juicy," where you want to linger.
- Rotate in the other direction.
- Do the other leg.

I don't have time for yoga!

Often when I am working with moms on yoga therapy, we make a plan, and then they come back in to see me and haven't done the practices. When you have a baby, you barely have time to pee, much less do yoga. When you are depressed, it can be hard to get started.

This is when it is really important to remember that yoga is not only what you see in a yoga class. Yoga does not have to be ninety minutes. Thirty will do. Five will do! Yoga does not have to involve doing any fancy poses, and in fact there are many formal yoga practices that you can do while you live your life, even while you are holding a baby in your arms.

This is a gift! For years before I had kids, I wished to have a home yoga practice. I would resolve to have a home practice but always failed to keep it up after about a week. Finding ninety minutes to go through a long sequence of poses was hard, and even when I had the time, I would often get distracted and give up halfway through. There's always an email to write, a phone call to answer, a dish to wash.

With pregnancy and with a baby, I had to make my goals much smaller. I couldn't do poses at all when I was sick and pregnant, and my first baby wanted to be held, in my arms, all the time. I learned that I could only practice every single day if I came up with practices that fit into my life as it was. And that stuck. I now practice yoga every day at home and at work. Sometimes it's a longer practice. Often it's one pose. Often it's a brief meditation or breath practice while waiting for something.

Let go, too, of needing a beautiful, quiet, or sacred place to practice. I think the most meaningful yoga practices I have ever done are on my mat in the middle of a kid mess, toys everywhere, maybe an episode of

Daniel Tiger on in the background as theme music, children climbing on my body every time I take a downward-facing dog pose.

One of the most basic yoga practices is mindfulness, or focusing on the present moment. You can practice mindfulness while you do everything and anything. You can nest mindfully, clean mindfully, breathe mindfully, love mindfully, birth mindfully, cry mindfully, and even fight mindfully. A teacher once told me you can do the dishes mindfully—I'm still working on that one.

It can be much less intimidating to develop a steady practice when we know that the practice can fit itself into our lives, instead of us having to contort our lives to meet the practice. You can make yoga contortion-free in every way!

Most of the practices in this book are meant to be doable with your baby, but here are a few practices you can easily do anywhere for just a few minutes, at any stage of pregnancy, postpartum, or life, and while holding a baby.

Practice **Mindful Awareness of This Moment in Pregnancy**

When you get the urge to look online to see "what to expect" in your body—slow it down. Consider spending that precious time that you would spend going down the rabbit hole of the Internet on feeling into your body instead.

- Notice what is happening now in your body.
- How does your body feel, in clothes, in the world?
- How do things smell?
- How do things taste? When you taste a food, experience it like it's your first time, letting go of stories about what you've liked before. Your taste buds may be working differently today. How does it taste now?

Practice **Breathing with Baby**

Breath practice is the easiest of all practices to do while holding a baby, as you have nowhere to go, and the breath is always there waiting for you.

Sit or stand with your baby. Bring your attention to your breath. Watch it rise and fall. You can also bring your attention to your baby's breath, noticing the difference in the rhythm of their breath and yours. When your mind wanders, gently bring it back.

Practice **Active Poses with Baby**

Here are some active poses you'll find elsewhere in this book that you can easily do with babe in arms or a carrier.

Baby in arms:
- Simple mindful movements (page 104)
- Warrior II pose (page 79)
- Tree pose (page 92)
- Lion's breath with wide squat (page 122)

Baby in a carrier:
- Rainbow arms and sun arms (page 197–198)
- Seated or standing side stretch (page 198)
- Standing chest stretch with wall (page 198)
- Keep-ups (page 117)

I'm having trouble bonding with my baby

Moms with PMADs, especially with depression, can have difficulty bonding or connecting with their babies. Moms may think:

- I know I am pregnant, but it's hard to feel it's an actual person in there.
- This baby feels like a stranger, like someone else's baby.
- Why don't I find my baby cute?
- I hate this baby for making me so miserable.
- I never felt the magical moment of falling in love that other moms describe.
- My baby dislikes me. She cries whenever I hold her.
- I am a terrible mother for feeling this way.

These thoughts are especially common in the early days, when your baby doesn't smile back, and cannot say "thank you," "I love you," or "I want . . . " Loving them may feel abstract, since you don't really know who they are yet.

A mom may shamefully or fearfully believe these thoughts are her whole truth. In my experience, however, most moms who feel this way do have a part of themselves that cares deeply for their baby—it's just that the depression is blocking their awareness of it.

I have watched mothers in my practice who thought they could never bond with their babies begin to fall deeply in love with them as they healed. One sign that a mom's depression is lifting? I see her eyes light up when her baby smiles at her or does something new, like roll over. I've seen this happen so many times that I have deep faith that love is always a possibility.

Patanjali's *Yoga Sutras*, Sutra 1.36, suggests that when distressed, you should focus on the "light within."[10] This is the light your yoga teacher mentions at the end of class when they say, "*Namaste*. The light in me honors the light in you." It's no hokey, New Age light or mere happiness described here—it's meant to be understood as the life force itself. What a reassuring idea—that even when we feel very disconnected, we can imagine and focus on a source of inner illumination, our own hearth, a force that ignites us.

I fell in love with this sutra when I heard it spoken by Jane Austin, my prenatal yoga teacher. "Each of us," she said, "has a light within. And when you are pregnant, you carry two lights inside of you!" (Or more, if you are carrying multiples!)

My heart skipped a beat when I heard this—I could imagine it, not only my own light, but the nascent light of my baby within. This was the beginning of our relationship, the first moment I bonded with my child, my older daughter whose light is now one of the most familiar I've known.

Even if you don't feel bonded with your baby or you struggle to connect to their light, you can help them form a healthy attachment to you. Have you ever heard the saying "Love is a verb"? Love doesn't have to be a fixed state. It can be found in behaviors, gestures of love. Acting as if you love your baby makes your baby feel loved.

A great way to offer a gesture of love to your baby, even if you don't feel it, is to use your voice. Babies really like to hear your voice. They can even hear your voice inside the womb. You might feel silly, but talking or singing to your baby, both in your belly and after they're born, stimulates them and helps them develop an attachment to your voice.

Often, when moms are depressed, they don't talk as much to their babies and they don't change the tone of their voice much—it's mostly monotone. When moms practice talking in a cheerful, varied tone to their babies, babies can become more securely attached.[11]

Practice Focus on the Light Within

To focus on your own light:
Sit, perhaps close your eyes, and imagine a light in your heart. Notice the color, shape, and brightness of the light. As you inhale, imagine it growing bigger, expanding to fill your whole body. As you exhale, imagine it drawing into its nucleus and becoming brighter. Repeat as long as you like.

To connect during pregnancy or with your baby:
Sit, perhaps closing your eyes. One hand can be on your belly (if pregnant), or your baby can be in your arms or right next to you. Imagine a light within your heart and another one within your baby's heart. As you inhale, imagine both lights growing bigger and connecting, entering each other's orbits, combining their brightness. As you exhale, imagine that they both draw back into their centers, two separate lights.

Practice Singing

Singing is a common yoga therapy practice, meant to uplift the soul. Singing calms your nervous system, as it involves long, steady exhales. Singing also provides that varied vocal tone we know is so good for babies. You do not need to sing on key for it to work!

Sing to your pregnant belly. Sing to your newborn as you hold them, feed them, change diapers, drive. It helps to have a "go-to" song. Find a song that is uplifting or meaningful to you. I like "Three Little Birds," by Bob Marley. Maybe there is a song from your faith tradition or a yoga chant you like.

You can also make a song up. This is especially fun for older babies and toddlers. Sing, "Now we are changing your diaper, now we are putting on shooooesss . . ." You can add rhymes or include their name. It can feel special to you and your child to have a song that is just yours. Making up songs is also a good mindfulness practice—being in the moment with whatever comes out of your mouth, letting go of judging how brilliant it is.

Constant change is hard

One of the hardest things about the perinatal time period is the diz-zying level of change—physical, mental, hormonal, identity. As soon as you feel like you understand something about your body or your baby, it changes.

First our energy levels change, then our preferences change—foods we used to find delicious suddenly repel us, and we develop cravings that might feel like they belong to someone else. Our shape changes. We get whole new wardrobes: maternity clothes, then post-baby clothes. We get stretch marks, our nipples change color, our feet grow, our hair gets thicker, and then hair falls out after we give birth.

Identity changes—people start to identify us as expecting moms. They talk to us differently, comment on our bodies, maybe even touch us. They don't ask us about our work or our love in the same way—they ask about the baby. Work changes. We shift goals and priorities; we face new questions: "What are you going to do with the baby?" "When are you going back to work?" Friendships change. We don't go out as much. Maybe we aren't as available to our friends. We may spend a lot of time with other people with kids, and it strains relation-ships with friends who don't have kids. Our relationships to our own parents change. Our relationship with our partner changes. Our sex drive changes. What feels good changes.

And then we have a child and the whole focus of life changes—our fears change, our preoccupations change, all of our daily activities change. Our child changes. Just as we get on our feet with one stage of parenting, our child has a developmental leap and changes again. And again. You master the art of baby swaddling just in time for your kiddo to worm out of it. You learn a magic calming song or what kind of bouncing soothes them just in time for them to pick a new song or type of bounce they like better.

Figuratively and literally, our center of gravity changes every day. This can be especially unsettling for those of us who struggle with anxiety, uncertainty, and lack of control. We can develop an urge to turn to compulsive behaviors to give us a sense of center, organizing and reorganizing our homes or regulating what we eat.

With all of these changes, it can become hard to know who we are! This experience can be a gift for our yoga practice, because it connects us to one of the most important tenets of yoga psychology—impermanence, the acknowledgment that nothing lasts forever. A breath comes and goes, thoughts come and go, feelings come and go, sensations come and go. Everything ages, every perfect moment ends, and, likewise, every challenge eventually passes. Though pregnancy may feel like forever, your baby is truly just a temporary visitor in your body. Our very lives are impermanent, coming and going. Practicing facing impermanence helps us let go of unhealthy attachments, accept change, and, most importantly, connect to what doesn't change—our true self, our pure awareness that resides before, during, and after all of this.

The good news is, even if you struggle to accept change, life is on your side. We don't have to seek out opportunities to let change happen—it just does. Life generously chips away at our attachments. All we have to do is notice.

Practice **Finding Your Center in Mountain Pose**

Start in mountain pose Stand with your feet about as far apart as your hip bones, or at a distance that lets you feel comfortable and steady, like an unmoving mountain. Invite the spine to be upright, and collarbones to broaden. Traditionally arms fall to the sides with palms facing forward. You can also do this with a baby in your arms or a carrier. Notice what it feels like to take this shape. What muscles hold you upright? Where do you feel your breath?

- Close your eyes.
- Slowly shift your weight to the left, noticing what muscles activate and compensate to keep you upright. Then slowly shift to the right, noticing.
- Find center, in between the two sides, noticing which muscles work and which muscles release. How do your bones align today in center?
- Slowly shift your weight forward, noticing, then shift back, noticing. Find center again, noticing.
- Sway slowly in a circle, then find center.

Notice, how do you feel when you are centered versus leaning?

Practice **Tree Pose**

Tree pose is a great place to practice meeting change. One day you might have finally "figured out" how to balance in tree pose with a pregnant belly. And then the next day your belly is even bigger and you have to learn it again. Then your baby is born and you have to adjust again to how to balance without the belly. Or how to balance with a baby in your arms.

- If you feel unsteady or are near the end of a pregnancy or holding a baby, be sure to be near a wall. You can keep one hand on the wall for support.
- Stand on one foot. Lift your other foot up and place it on the inside of the calf or thigh (just not the knee). Your hands can meet at the center of the chest, palms together, or can reach up into the sky like branches. Find your balance.

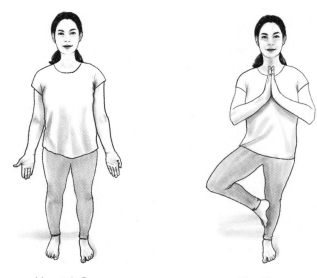

Mountain Pose   Tree Pose

Notice that there is no stillness in this pose. To stay upright, you must continually make micromovements, readjusting your balance in tiny ways, using different muscles. I like to think about how this is like real trees. Trees that are flexible and can sway in the wind don't get knocked over. If a tree becomes brittle, it is more likely to get pushed down by the wind.

I need help

You cannot recover alone. Healing requires connection. Self-care can feel burdensome or hollow if we don't get support from others. Seeing a therapist who works with new moms, who can offer you knowledge, compassion, and guidance, can be a life raft. Gathering our community close and maintaining friendships can sustain us through our darkest times.

Unfortunately, there are many barriers to asking for help. You may not have much help available. Finances or insurance may be an obstacle to getting professional help. Maybe you just moved, or all your friends have babies, too. Maybe you have a painful relationship with your own family, so you don't want to reach out to them. You may fear judgment or being a burden, or fear letting others hold the baby.

Sometimes, our world becomes so small, so focused on baby, survival, and worries, that we ignore our community. They may feel alienated and unsure about whether we still love them or how they could reach out. Disconnect begets disconnect.

Worse, PMADs are invisible. No one can read your mind or know that you are suffering. And if they don't know you are suffering, they may not reach out to help.

When I was depressed and very exhausted with a new baby, I felt as if my face were distorted. It felt stiff and heavy, and like it didn't quite work right. I sometimes felt as if I were wearing thick glasses smeared with Vaseline. I'd smile and it would feel false and strange. I thought often that I must seem gloomy or socially awkward.

Strangely, friends would tell me how beautiful and glowing I was. I heard more than once that motherhood "suited" me. When I look back at pictures, I see that my smile looks perfectly normal, even lovely. Suffering doesn't write itself on one's face.

When you are in the latter part of your pregnancy, your body is very visible, and people may rush to help you carry something or give you their seat. But they don't always offer to visit, to make you food, to check in on how you are doing. And once the baby is born, most of their focus goes to the baby.

Practicing *satya*, truthfulness or honesty, with people in your life can help them help you. It might also be a gift for them: people love to feel needed and trusted.

This is especially true in intimate relationships. Partners of people with PMADs often feel very lost about how to help. They may struggle to acknowledge what is happening with you because they do not understand it, because it is painful to think about, or because they, too, are struggling with exhaustion, overwhelm, and identity changes. They may have tried to help a few times, but feel like everything they try is wrong—nothing helps. They may also take your sadness, rage, or anxiety personally and feel rejected, frustrated, confused, helpless, or angry. They may feel lonely if you are not able to connect with them like you used to.

I have often heard partners say things like, "I want my wife back." I always feel frustrated when I hear this because I think, *Your wife is right here! She is just suffering or sick right now. She needs you to see her whole self.* This is why honest communication about your feelings and needs is so important. Not only does honesty help you heal, but it also helps your relationship. Your partner needs to know and see both the healthy and suffering parts of you. They need to know your truth so that they can grow and develop skills to in order to support you.

Do not worry about being a burden—it will only be a burden if you hold your feelings inside, and your partner feels left alone. In those traditional wedding vows, when they talk about "in sickness and health"? This is "in sickness." Relationships are not only for happy people. The beauty of a relationship is how it can hold you through both ups and downs.

It helps to remember that asking your partner—or anyone, for that matter—for help doesn't mean you are giving them the burden of fixing you. You don't need to be fixed, but you probably do need to feel loved as you are. Maybe you just need them to hold your hand or give you long hugs. Maybe you need to commiserate and connect on how both of you are struggling together. Maybe you need someone to listen and ask good questions. And be clear with them: articulating what kind of help you need doesn't mean your partner has to be the one to fulfill it, especially if they are overwhelmed too. It might mean that they collaborate with you on how to find and support you in using outside resources.

If you have a partner, consider reminding yourself often that you are just that—partners, a team, a family. What helps you helps the whole team. Notice if you get caught up in resentments, shame, blame, or scorekeeping ("I got up twice with the baby last night, and you only got up once.") If you are both on the same team, you share points.

Instead, focus on connecting, collaborating, problem solving, and caring for one another as you navigate this trying time. Help educate your partner about what you need. If you don't know, you can work on figuring it out together. Couples therapy or individual therapy for partners can also be supportive for you and your "team."

Practice **Honesty with Friends and Family**

Here are some things you can tell your friends and family. Feel free to just hand them this chapter (and cross off whichever things don't apply to you, or add on things I missed).

I am struggling with depression and/or anxiety.

I can be struggling even when I look very put together.

I need lots of warmth, support, and encouragement.

Encourage me to rest and get more sleep, but also help me figure out how I can do that—it feels frustrating if you tell me to rest when I don't know who will help me out.

Offer to take a night shift.

Encourage me to eat regularly. Bring nourishing food or get a group of friends to bring meals.

When you visit, offer to take care of the baby so I can lie down. I will protest and say I want to hang out with you. Insist I go lie down or take a shower. Tell me you will hang out with me another time.

Clean up three things in my house.

Drive me to an appointment.

Invite me out for a walk and help me get out the door.

Don't ask me what I need in an open-ended way. I'll be overwhelmed and tell you I don't need anything. Offer what you can do and then make sure it's okay with me. Try saying, "I'm bringing you a meal and dropping it on your doorstep at 5 p.m. Is that okay? I'm happy to come inside and say hi or just to leave it."

Don't tell me to focus on how lucky I am or how beautiful the baby is. Don't tell me not to worry. Validate what's hard, offer compassion, tell me you see how much I am struggling. If you've been through it, let me know that you understand. Make lots of space for my feelings.

Offer to hold my baby for a few minutes so I can practice yoga. Offer to sit quietly in meditation with me for five minutes. Accept it if I tell you I'm not in the mood for yoga today.

Tell me that anything I need to do to be well is okay. Don't lecture me on the importance of being all natural, or suggest my problems will be fixed by following a specific diet or even doing yoga.

If I don't want to spend money on therapy, yoga, or a babysitter, tell me to let that go. Tell me this is not a time for saving; this is a time for investing in my family.

If I don't have financial resources, help me find low-fee services.

Give me as little advice as possible and as much love as possible.

Let me know I don't have to get worse to be taken seriously.

Trust I will get through this with support. Be patient and have faith.

Get some support yourself. It's hard to see a loved one or friend suffer.

Remember I am grateful to you for being here for me. Thank you.

Section Two
Welcome and Move with Your Thoughts and Feelings

Depression and anxiety bring with them crashing waves of difficult thoughts and feelings. You might feel exhausted, frazzled, sad, angry, numb, or overwhelmed. You might wonder how you can survive these emotions and how you can be a parent in the midst of them. In this section, you will explore how to welcome and cope with painful thoughts and feelings. You will learn that you do not need to force yourself to be calm, grateful, blissful, or happy. You can bring your most difficult feelings with you as you move through your day, honoring them, letting your body find movement with them, letting yourself be in stillness with them. You will learn how to choose the type of yoga practice that fits the thoughts and feelings that arise, helping you shift your energy and find solace, strength, and center.

I just want to feel better

If you've ever been in therapy, you've probably been told that you have to "sit with your feelings."

My experience as a therapist is that when I talk to people about sitting with feelings, they roll their eyes, tell me that it doesn't work, and generally start to get even more agitated. Feelings are hard—who on earth would want to sit with them? People just want to feel better.

There is also something about "sitting with feelings" that implies stuckness, paralysis, lack of doing something to feel better. And the perinatal period is already filled with experiences of stuckness. When you are pregnant, you are stuck with that baby inside of you for a long time. In labor, when you decide you change your mind because this hurts too much? Sorry—you are stuck getting that baby out one way or another. With your little one, when you want to sleep more than anything you've ever wanted to do before? You are stuck sitting with them—or rather, bouncing with them, all night long. It's pretty natural that you may not like it if I suggest that you now choose to sit and be stuck with your feelings, too.

Instead of sitting with feelings, in yoga therapy we talk about "welcoming feelings." If we welcome feelings, we are not stuck, we can bring them along with us as we move through life. We can find spaciousness and expansiveness around them. We don't have to waste energy holding onto them or pushing them away.

Welcoming feelings can be terrifying. Some of us experience difficult feelings in our bodies as pain, restlessness, or tension. We might worry that if we welcome our feelings, they will never go away. They will grow too strong and destroy us. We believe we must resist them. Others may warn us, too, that we need to "just let go" or "get over it." We may tell ourselves that welcoming or even allowing feelings means we are being negative, living in fear, giving in to depression or anxiety, or being lazy.

Maddeningly, the more we try to make feelings go away, the louder they get. Have you ever had a mosquito bite? The itch of a mosquito bite can be unbearable, and there is nothing on earth you want to do more than scratch it to make the itch go away. The frustrating part is, the more you scratch, the worse the itching gets. A salve or itch cream can help a little, but it doesn't make it go away. The only real way to make the itch go away is to let the itch be and stop scratching long enough to let your body heal on its own. With feelings, we can soothe ourselves or avoid them as much as we want to, but at some point, we have to let them run their course.

If letting them run their course sounds awful, the good news is that we can benefit from listening to our feelings. Sometimes feelings make a lot of sense and point us to needs. Sadness may tell us that we have lost something valuable, and need to shore ourselves up. Anxiety may tell us we need more grounding. Anger may tell us that we need to stand up for ourselves. Other times, feelings follow faulty thoughts, and we need to open our minds up to seeing things more clearly. We can't learn any of these insights about ourselves if we simply say that we "shouldn't" feel something.

Welcoming feelings is the rich work of witnessing ourselves, of letting go of what we should feel and seeing honestly what we do feel, of experiencing ourselves as open, expansive awareness that can truly hold so much.

If we open ourselves up to our emotions, we can begin to see that feelings come and go, often rising like a wave, and then slowly falling. We can see that we can actually move through our lives with them—no need to stop everything until they go away. You can take your worry with you to go meet another mom for a playdate. You can take your rage with you on a walk. You can take your self-hatred to the grocery store. You can take your despair with you to work, and you can kiss your baby in the midst of the deepest suffering.

Practice Welcoming Feelings and Finding Spaciousness

Before you can welcome feelings, you have to know what they are. This seems like it should be easy, but it can actually be difficult. Most of the time when I ask moms what they are feeling, they say "I feel like I need some sleep" or "I feel like I'm doing a terrible job." These are not feelings—they are thoughts!

Feelings can be labeled with one word, like sadness, anger, fear, joy, or calm. So "I feel like I need some sleep" might truly be "I feel overwhelmed" and "I feel like I'm doing a terrible job" might be, "I feel ashamed."

Take a moment to turn inward and explore a difficult emotion that is salient for you right now, perhaps one that you want to make go away.

Ask yourself,

"What is this feeling?
What is its name? (Label it with a feeling word.)
Where and how do I feel it in my body?
What thoughts come up around it?
What stories or memories emerge?
What urges do I have around this feeling?"

When you notice your mind seeking to fix or avoid the feeling, practice saying "Welcome" to the feeling inside your mind. Notice if your breath stopped or became shallow, and perhaps experiment with letting it be deep and full again. Notice if your body became tense or rigid around the feeling, and, if it feels right, let it soften.

Sadness

Moms with PMADs often feel sad. Sometimes sadness feels like it has an obvious cause—sadness about missing your old life, sadness about how hard things are for you, sadness about something that happened in your relationships or at work, sadness about feeling left alone with your baby. Other times the sadness is just there, and you find yourself crying for no particular reason.

What does sadness feel like in your body? In yoga therapy, sadness is thought to have a quality called *tamas*, which roughly translates to darkness—bringing heaviness, fogginess, inertia, obstruction, exhaustion, and ignorance of our true divine nature. When this quality becomes quite strong, it can also lead to depression. Some signs that this quality has set in might be:

- Sleeping too much
- Overeating
- Feelings of worthlessness and hopelessness
- Thoughts like *I can't do this—it's too hard.*
- Difficulty doing daily tasks

When you feel heavy, stuck, and depressed, you might notice that you become stiff or slumped, curled into yourself. You may feel flat or numb, or have a feeling that you aren't truly alive.

Your body is born knowing how to welcome this stuck feeling and move it through you: by crying. But by the time we reach our teen years, most of us learn to resist crying. We tense our faces to keep tears in. We apologize for our tears. We tell ourselves it's stupid or ugly or weak to cry. We put our hands over our face, to hide tears. We grab a tissue right away, as though we could wipe away our emotions. The emotions, then, stay inside, and the stuck feeling grows.

Sometimes, crying doesn't help—we could cry for days, and it just makes us more stuck and sad. Other times, it's only when we surrender to crying and just let ourselves bawl that sadness can flow through. If we really let it run its course without criticizing ourselves, even if it means crying for hours, we might notice afterward that we feel a bit clearer, less dark, and less heavy. If we let ourselves cry in front of someone else, we might feel more seen and more loved. The sadness will likely still be there, but it may not be as devastating. We may even get insight into what needs lie beneath it—like connecting with community, or expressing ourselves through art or talking to a friend.

In yoga therapy, we try to do the same thing with movement. We can invite ourselves to notice this heavy, stuck feeling, welcome it in, and move with it. We don't force it out, but we also don't let it pull us down into inertia. We can move with it in our lives—continuing to go out, connect with others, take a shower. We can also move with it in our asana practice. If big movements seem out of the question, we can focus on smaller movements that just break up a little of the heaviness, as if we were the tin man, lubricating our joints with an oil can.

Practice **Simple Mindful Movements**

Simple mindful movements, when combined with breath and attention, are powerful medicine for depression, freeing up stuck energy and increasing vitality. They can reduce physical stiffness and discomfort, increase flexibility and range of motion, and invite a deeper breath. They are accessible and unintimidating when exhausted, and they do not require strength, a mat, or any special clothes. You can even do them in bed. They can be practiced at any stage of pregnancy or with a baby in your lap.

Here is a series of simple dynamic movements you might like to try. You can do just one, do them all, or make up some of your own. Move in sync with the breath. You may want to play with exhaling as you close a joint, inhaling as you open it. I recommend that you do each movement five times before you move on to another one. This sequence can be done on the floor or in a chair.

Feet Point the toes. Then flex the feet.

Ankles Rotate the ankles.

Knees Bend the knee. Then straighten the leg. If on the floor, you may want to use your hands to help lift the leg up so it has room to bend.

Hips If on the floor, you can come onto hands and knees. In a chair, stay seated. Lift the right knee up about an inch. Slowly make little circles with the knee in one direction and then the other. If it feels good, you may want to move on to making big circles with the knee, opening the hip all the way out to the side as you go. Then do the other leg.

Spine 1 (seated) Put hands on knees, lengthen spine, and arch chest forward into a gentle backbend. Then round the spine forward, letting head fall; press front body into back body.

Spine 2 (hands and knees) This is like cat/cow on page 165. On hands and knees, inhale as you look forward and arch the chest into a small backbend. On the exhale, round the spine, looking in at your belly. Do this for a few rounds.

Spinal twist Sitting or standing upright, exhale and gently let the left shoulder twist you toward the left. Inhale center. Exhale and gently let the right shoulder twist you toward the right. Let this be very gentle, not using head or hands to wrench you deeply into the twist in either direction.

Shoulder circles Bring hands to the shoulders and draw circles with the elbows in one direction and then the other, rotating the shoulders in their sockets.

Wrists With arms straight, circle wrists in one direction, then the other.

Fingers Make a fist, then open hands out wide, spreading fingers straight.

Head Rotate your head in a semicircle, ear toward shoulder to chin toward chest, to other ear toward shoulder.

Jaw Take a big yawn.

Anxiety, fear, and panic

Another common emotion moms may struggle with is anxiety—and its sister emotions, fear and panic.

What does anxiety feel like in your body? In yoga therapy, anxiety is thought to have a quality called *rajas,* or activation. Activation brings agitation, friction, relentlessness, irritability, turbulence, and distraction. This activating energy is responsible for fantasy and imagination. And persistent negative fantasy, which we usually call worry, is the key symptom of the Western understanding of anxiety.

This idea of anxiety as activating energy maps on well to how our nervous system works. When our body perceives threat, our sympathetic nervous system (SNS) turns on to help us find safety. You might have heard this called the "fight, flight, or freeze" response. Your heart rate increases, your breath becomes shallow and fast, your muscles tense up, you sweat, and your digestion slows, causing your mouth to feel dry. These are all useful things if you're scared because you are running away from a bear.

Unfortunately, our body is a bit of a one-hit-wonder when it comes to dealing with stressful situations. Our SNS only does this one "fight, flight, or freeze" response. So it does the same thing when you worry that your baby might come into contact with germs as it does when the bear is chasing you. You can activate your SNS with thoughts alone. When you have an anxiety disorder, your body can become exhausted from spending so much time in this state of activation.

Some signs that your PMAD has the quality of activation include:

- Difficulty sleeping
- Loss of appetite
- Persistent worries

- Fantasies about bad things happening
- Difficulty letting go of tasks, or thoughts like *If I slow down or take a moment to rest, I will never get anything done*
- Preoccupation with keeping your house or your surroundings clean
- Difficulty doing daily tasks because worries get in the way

Just as with stuck energy of sadness, our bodies are designed to work through and release activating energy. In a more primal state, we would actually fight or flee! Big body movements like punching, kicking, shaking, or running put the hormones that the SNS releases to good use.

Most of us, especially girls and women, have been socialized to try to be calm, compliant, and nice, and to avoid these big expressions of feeling and releases of energy. We have learned that if someone feels anxious, they should simply "let it go," "just relax," or "calm down." But when an anxiety disorder is present, trying to "just relax" can be torture.

I often recommend to exhausted clients of mine that they do restorative yoga poses. But if I recommend that to someone with anxiety? They come back and tell me that restful poses made things worse, that they lay there feeling agitated and annoyed, or perhaps their minds sped up, offering a bevy of worries. Being told to relax can also be triggering for those with trauma histories, who were told to relax during their trauma, or for those who had anxiety earlier in life and had caretakers who dismissed them, leaving them alone with their fears.

What usually works better is actually inviting our anxious body to do what it would do in nature—move with the feeling. Going for a walk or a run can sometimes help. A dynamic yoga practice that involves big movements can also sometimes help you work through anxious energy. Then perhaps, at the end of your practice, you will have released some anxiety and be able to have a soothing rest in savasana or seated meditation. Maybe you will emerge feeling ready to face things you have been avoiding.

Practice Move with Your Anxiety

Here is an active sequence, designed to burn through overactive energy.

Start by telling yourself that you do not have to be calm, nor do you need to evaluate the effectiveness of this practice based on whether you still feel anxious afterward. The aim is not to make anxiety go away; it is to move with it. This is all about willingness—willingness to let the feeling be there. If you moved while feeling anxious, you've done the practice successfully.

I suggest beginning standing up, to help you embrace the idea that you do not need to relax.

Mountain pose (page 91)

Standing side stretch (page 198)

Standing dynamic twists—feet a little bit wider than hip-distance apart, knees slightly bent, swing your torso from side to side, letting your arms fly passively as you move

Forward fold (page 187)

Downward-facing dog or sun salutations (page 223)

Dynamic warrior II—Exhale into a Warrior II stance, as described on page 79. As you inhale, straighten the front knee and lift the arms to the sky, activating the muscles strongly by imagining that you are moving them through water. Exhale back to warrior II, again activating the muscles in the arms by pushing them down, as though through water.

Chair pose (page 179)

Wave squats (page 132)

Child's pose (page 200)

Savasana/final resting pose (page 128)

I can't stop worrying!

When we are feeling depressed or anxious, our tendency is often to think many steps ahead. In psychology we call this type of worry "fortune-telling" or "future-tripping." When you are pregnant, it's easy for this tendency to go on overdrive. Because you can't see or touch your baby, all your mind can do is create fantasies about who they will be. You might picture what your baby's hair might be like, what adventures you will go on together—maybe what it will be like at their high school graduation or when they become an adult. Until your child is an adult, this type of fantasizing is hard to avoid.

When you are depressed or anxious, however, these types of predictions can take a sinister turn. If your baby doesn't move in your pregnant belly, you might anxiously imagine them dying. When your one-month-old doesn't sleep, you might fear they will never sleep through the night and you will suffer for years on end. If your baby gets a fever, you might convince yourself that they have a serious illness.

If you express these snowballing thoughts out loud, friends listening to you might say, "Don't think like that—that's ridiculous." You might even hear yourself say, "I know this is irrational, but . . . " On a bad day, you might even get mad at yourself, saying, "I know this is stupid to think about, but I guess I'm stupid; I can't stop it."

If, instead of judging ourselves for irrational thoughts, we notice in a kind and curious way, we can begin to watch and learn how our thoughts turn into a runaway train. We can practice slowing ourselves down and stopping the train of thoughts when it goes off the rails. We can notice, *Wow, I'm really fortune-telling here. My worries are getting ahead of me.* This frees you up to seek out evidence, outside perspectives, and information, or practice sitting with the reality of uncertainty.

Yoga and mindfulness practices are like weight lifting for your mind, slowly strengthening your ability to notice thoughts and slow them down. When you start lifting weights, you don't start by lifting 200 pounds. You start small—maybe even with three-pound weights. It takes lots of practice to more easily notice and let go of thought distortions.

Practice **Just This Inhale**

Sometimes, especially when we're depressed or anxious, even focusing on the breath in meditation is a big ask. I've had days when I truly couldn't rein my mind in to watch an entire in-breath and out-breath, much less several breaths in a row. It's easy to get frustrated and stop meditating.

On days like this, "just this inhale" is a good place to start. Expectations are moderate, and chances of success are high. Just one inhale can bring a moment of peace, ease, and focus.

Start by releasing the idea that your mind must be clear. Then release any ideas you have that you are supposed to follow your breath for any length of time.

Take a deep, slow breath, focusing on JUST THIS INHALE. Notice what it feels like in your body—in your nose, your chest, and your belly. Notice the edges of just this inhale—the moment of emptiness at the beginning and the moment of fullness as you crest toward the exhale. Resist a pull to notice anything else. If your mind begins to wander, you might tell it, "Hang on—I will follow that train of thought in one second—I'm just following this one inhale, and it's almost done."

You can do this for only one breath, right when you need it most, in a moment of anger, exhaustion, boredom, or overwhelm. You can also allow it to morph into a longer seated meditation. That can feel great, but you've already succeeded if you only notice one inhale.

Preoccupations

Certain kinds of worries, rather than snowballing, seem to be like a scratched record. They repeat and repeat in our minds. In psychology, we call these thoughts preoccupations or obsessions. Common preoccupations include worries about:

- Health—yours, your partner's, or the baby's
- Safety—yours, your partner's, or the baby's
- Cleanliness, germs, and toxic substances
- Harm or something bad happening to the baby
- Forgetting the baby somewhere, dropping the baby, molesting the baby, or hurting the baby

A majority of new moms have scary thoughts like this. They help us heighten our awareness of threat and protect our babies. But when anxiety or OCD is present, as may be the case when we're struggling with PMADs, the thoughts get sticky and hard to let go of or see through. We might do something to make sure that our babies are healthy or safe, like go to a doctor's appointment or have a professional check our car seat installation, but these actions somehow don't provide relief—the worries are still there.

The hard thing about some of these preoccupations is that, unlike fortune-telling worries, it's hard to point to them as distortions. Some of these things actually could happen, even though they probably won't. Yes, your baby could get sick or die, you could get in an accident, you could have lead in your paint, you could forget your baby in the back of the car.

What most of us do when we have thoughts like this is try to reassure ourselves that these things will not happen. We may try to do research on the Internet, reading everything we can about what illnesses our baby might have, what terrible things could happen, and how to prevent them. We might ask family or friends to promise us that these bad things won't happen. The problem with this pattern—which, in psychology, we call "reassurance seeking"—is that it often only makes anxiety worse.

If you find one website that tells you that your baby probably doesn't have whatever disease you are researching, you may feel like you need to check another one. If your partner reassures you, you may think they just don't get it, they are not worried enough, and you can't trust them now. Plus, if someone reassures you that some awful thing just wouldn't happen, they've inadvertently reinforced the idea that the feared situation is as awful as you believed. The more you try to make preoccupations go away, the stronger they get.

In yoga, this cycle is known as *abhinivesha*, meaning fear of death, and it is described as one of the great afflictions, or *kleshas*, of humans. We are told that the path to overcoming the great afflictions is to study them in ourselves, meditate on them, and face them with dedication.

Yoga therapy and psychology share wisdom on this situation—psychology calls this process of facing our feared thoughts "exposure." Exposure is one of the most effective ways to deal with fears and preoccupations.

Practice **Meditating on Difficult Thoughts**

Facing difficult thoughts can be just that—difficult. If your preoccupations are only mildly bothersome, you can do this practice on your own. If that feels overwhelming, you can do this work with a therapist.

Pick a preoccupation that disturbs you, such as "My child could get the flu."

- Say to yourself:

These fears are thoughts. They are anxiety—preoccupations.
I am not going to reassure myself; that just perpetuates the fear.
*   I am willing to feel my fear and anxiety.*
Yes, this thing could happen.

- Invite the thought in.
- Try repeating it over and over. Maybe say it out loud.
- Bask in the thought, and try to hold onto it—if your mind wanders, come right back to it.
- Notice what happens within you as you hold this thought—how feelings may rise and fall like waves. Notice urges to reassure yourself and go back to the thought.
- Maybe experiment with imagining what would happen if your fear came true. What would it be like? What would you do?

At the end of your meditation, it might help to take time to come back to the present moment. You might try moving your body a little bit, taking in the room around you, perhaps noticing colors or objects around you. After your meditation, resist the urge to go right into reassuring-seeking behaviors. You might even tell loved ones that if you start asking them again if your fears are true, that they should gently refuse to reassure you, and offer you love instead.

What if I can't stand this physical discomfort?

Most moms experience some serious discomfort while pregnant. Nausea, heartburn, back pain, swollen feet, and that impatient feeling at the end when you just want that baby out. Labor brings intense pain, and often, fear and anticipation of that pain ahead of time is the most uncomfortable part. Even if you plan to get an epidural, you cannot avoid all pain—you will likely go through contractions before you get to the epidural. You might find the epidural itself painful. Recovering from childbirth and early breastfeeding can be painful. You may find yourself sleeping in a weird position, shoulder smushed and aching, trying not to move so you don't wake your baby up.

In yoga, we often hold poses that bring strong sensations that we might think we can't stand. While they do not simulate anywhere near the level of pain experienced in childbirth, they can provide insight into how your mind reacts when you face something extremely unpleasant, be it a contraction, a baby crying, or even a challenging emotion.

Keep-ups, yoga arm holds from the Kundalini tradition, are among the most useful and accessible of the challenging yoga practices for the perinatal time period. Keep-ups are often taught in prenatal yoga classes as birth preparation. This is where I was first introduced to them, in my teacher Jane's class. In keep-ups, you hold your arms up for a long time—up to eleven minutes! Keep-ups seem like simple poses, but as you hold them, strong sensations arise in the arms and the mind can become restless.

My experience from teaching keep-ups in my prenatal yoga classes is that most minds begin with this thought:

What is this? It doesn't seem like regular yoga. It seems too simple. It's not giving me enough exercise. It is silly.

And then, once it gets challenging, minds might say:

This is so awful. I cannot do this. I need to put my arms down. Why is she teaching us this? This is crazy! When will this end? I cannot stand it.

Or:

I have to prove how good I am by holding my arms up the entire time. I will not put them down no matter what. Holding up my arms means I am strong, a good mother, and I'll be awesome at labor.

Often people have all of these thoughts simultaneously.

With regular practice, moms learn what thought waves to expect, and what kind of breath or self-talk they need in order to stay with it. Many moms have told me that this self-knowledge is the most helpful yoga tool they have in labor and the first months of motherhood. They tell me that they remember the fortitude they built in keep-ups to stay with themselves in the moments in labor when they wanted to give up. They tell me that they draw on that strength, too, at that 3 a.m. awakening, when they can't put their crying baby down.

I have found they are also useful for dealing with a toddler! When my daughter was three, she had a book called *The Knuffle Bunny* (get it, it's cute!) and wanted to read it over and over and over. I would start to feel bored, frustrated, restless. I would want to scream, "I'm not reading it anymore!" I judged myself for not being more patient, fun, or present, for being too selfish to just enjoy, something my daughter so obviously loved.

I realized one day that what my mind did in keep-ups was exactly like what it did during the book. Knowing what I needed to get through the keep-ups helped me get through the book. Book time got easier. Eventually my daughter forgot the book and moved on to a new one, proving that nothing with kids lasts forever.

Practice **Keep-ups**

- Hold up arms out to your sides in a pose of receptivity, hands open, elbows bent, hands at shoulder height.
- Soften your shoulders.
- Find your breath.
- Notice what your mind does.
- See how you can soften and deepen your breath to stay with it.

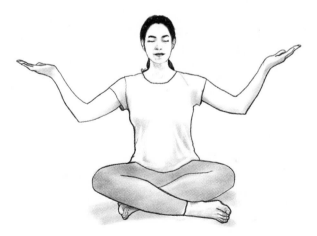

Keep-ups

You can try these things to help yourself stay with it:

- Tell yourself "I can do it" instead of "I have to do it."
- Acknowledge it is hard.
- Smile at how human your reaction is.
- See if you can last three breaths longer than your mind says you can.
- Tell yourself that it's okay to pause, but come back as soon as you are ready.
- Use your breath.
- Notice an urge to criticize or force yourself to stay with it. Can you let go? Can you cheerlead without criticism?
- Notice pain, breathe awareness into the fullness of the pain, and then exhale awareness into the center of the pain.
- Reassure yourself that nothing bad is going to happen. There are many yoga poses that can injure you if you approach them too fiercely— this is not one of them. You cannot injure yourself with keep-ups.
- Focus attention on parts of your body that can be totally at ease, like the soles of your feet, your forehead, or your tongue.

I recommend starting with three minutes and work up to five. Once you can do five, consider doing two sets.

Rage

Some moms with PMADs never notice feeling sad or anxious, but instead experience rage. Sometimes, rage is seething, leaving you annoyed and irritable. Other times, rage bursts to the surface, bringing an urge to yell or do something violent. Angry urges are common when you feel exhausted or depressed, and you are not alone. You haven't suddenly become a mean, always angry person—this is a symptom of PMADs, and you need and deserve support to get through it.

You may have legitimate things to be angry about: maybe your partner left you with too much of the work. Maybe your community let you down by not providing enough support. Maybe your doctor said something hurtful. Having anger is not a sign of pathology or selfishness—it's a normal human emotion. When we are not depressed, we can marshal anger into effective action, advocating for ourselves, communicating effectively, setting boundaries, or joining with community to make changes.

When we are depressed or anxious, however, anger can get stuck in a painful cycle of blame and shame. We might have ruminative thoughts about how others let us down. Even sharing feelings and thoughts doesn't feel like enough, and expressions of rage tend to escalate, which might make loved ones angry right back at us. We might feel ashamed about our rage, turning it in on ourselves, and then back at our loved ones.

When you're angry, avoid saying things to yourself like, "You are upsetting the baby and ruining your family. Get yourself together. Just relax. This isn't a big deal. Just go do yoga and you'll feel better." There are few things in life less relaxing than someone saying, "Just relax." Yoga doesn't work that way, and this is a set-up for thinking, *Yoga doesn't work*. Practiced over time, yoga helps you develop "muscles" of self-observation, emotional regulation, compassion, and clarity. You get better at saying things to yourself like:

- I notice I'm feeling angry.
- I notice how my body feels.
- This is a human emotion.
- Everyone feels angry sometimes.
- Even good moms get angry.
- Upsetting thoughts can color the way I see things. I might have a more nuanced view of this when my thoughts and my body are calmer.
- I have an urge to do something I might regret later.
- I notice this, and I have some choice right now.
- This anger is expressing a need, perhaps to feel better or to be heard.
- I can find a good way to meet my need.
- I can take a break.
- I can use my yoga practice to support me.
- If my anger is too intense for yoga, I can do something else, like scream into a pillow, write an angry "unsent" letter, or run very cold or warm water over my hands.
- I can ride the wave of this emotion. It may get more intense for a little bit, but it won't last forever.
- I will get through this.

Imagine that your rage is a wave. Avoid confrontations at the top of the wave. At the height of anger, we have a hard time listening, and we may trigger others to get angry back at us. This makes it hard for them to truly listen to us and/or consider changing. It's always a good idea to take a break and come back to talk when your wave of anger has subsided. In a fit of anger you might say to the other person, "I love you and care about our relationship. I am really angry right now, and I don't want to say or do something out of anger. I need a break. Let's talk about this when I'm calmer."

If you have an overwhelming urge to scream at, or in front of, your baby or to shake your baby, please know that it is much better to leave your baby, alone for a moment, even if they are crying. Put them in a safe place, like their crib. Go to another room or outside for a moment. Breathe. Do whatever it takes to slow yourself down, whether it's noticing how you are feeling and talking yourself through it, doing some sun salutations (page 223), screaming into a pillow, or using lion's breath (on the next page). Come back. You didn't hurt them. You did a really good job. If you feel ready, pick your baby up and give some cuddles. Sometimes that cuddle is soothing for both of you when you return.

Once you ride out a wave of rage, you may find that sadness or exhaustion set in. This is a good time to seek out soothing and kindness, to ask yourself what needs lie underneath the anger.

Practice **Lion's Breath**

Lion's breath can be useful to let out some immediate steam. Open your eyes as wide as you can, stick your tongue out as far as you can, and allow your face to become quite fierce with rage. Take a big loud exhale, like the sound Darth Vader makes.

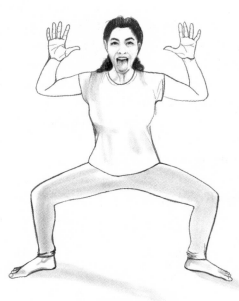

Lion's Breath

If you have arms and legs free, you can add full body movement. Stand with your feet wide. As you inhale, reach your arms up in the air. As you exhale into your lion's breath, bend your elbows, and pull your arms down with your fingers spread very wide while lowering your seat into a wide standing squat. Inhale back to the initial position and repeat a few more times if you like.

Sometimes I wonder if this was all a mistake

When new moms come into my office, they often tell me, in a hushed voice, a thought they feel deeply ashamed of, usually with a caveat of "I know this is awful, but . . . sometimes I wonder if this was all a mistake," they say, or "I wish I had never gotten pregnant," or "I should never have become a mother," or "I sometimes hate or resent my baby."

These thoughts are so painful because she thinks that she isn't supposed to have them. She thinks she is the only mother who has them. She thinks that having these thoughts means she cannot also love her child. Maybe she has been afraid to say them out loud for fear that makes them more true. She tries to push these thoughts away, and they just come back stronger.

She might feel especially ashamed for having these thoughts if she had a hard time getting pregnant, if she has a history of miscarriage or loss, or if she used fertility medicine or in vitro fertilization (IVF). She may also feel ashamed if a close friend or family member is struggling to have a child. She asks, "How could I feel these things when I wanted this baby so much?" "How could I resent my child when I am so lucky to have one?"

What she is experiencing is ambivalence, which can be a deeply normal and healthy part of motherhood. Ambivalence means we hold two opposite emotions toward the same thing. When we rigidly hold ourselves to one emotion, rejecting the other, ambivalence turns into pathology, and at worst, we find ourselves acting a bit unconsciously. For example, if we allow ourselves to express only gratitude and joy about having our babies, we might find ourselves acting out our resentment toward them in ways we don't understand—like fearing our baby hates us, or that our baby will grow up to be evil—or even having suicidal or homicidal thoughts.

But we do not need to hold ourselves to one emotion! Just because you express a complaint doesn't mean you are not grateful. Just because you are pregnant and wish you didn't have swollen feet or swollen boobs or acid reflux doesn't mean you don't love your future kiddo. Just because you sometimes don't want to be a mom doesn't mean that being a mom isn't what you want more than anything. Just because you really want to go back to work doesn't mean you don't also wish you could be home with your baby. Just because you appreciate your partner doesn't mean you don't want to throw them out the window when they leave a towel on the floor. You can love and hate someone at the same time—in fact, you probably can't really love someone without sometimes hating them.

When we make room for ambivalence, when we are willing to welcome and live with these opposites, we can experience the fullness, the messiness of what it means to be alive. We can wake up to our true nature, our ground of being, unchanging awareness that welcomes everything. Holding opposites is the gateway into true mental and spiritual flexibility and health.

We do not need to worry that feelings of ambivalence mean that we are going to do something bad. Feelings are not actions. They can lead to actions, especially when we don't have awareness of them. We can always choose our actions based on what is important to us, what we value, and what we truly believe is best.

Practice Opposite Emotions Meditation

As you sit or lie in meditation, notice an emotion that you are experiencing or that you want to explore. Invite that emotion in. Feel it in your body, noticing sensations. If images or thoughts come up, notice that, too.

Now ask yourself what an opposite emotion might be. There is no wrong answer, just something that makes sense to you. Invite that emotion in. If it's hard to access, try recalling a time when you felt that emotion. Feel it in your body, or imagine feeling it in your body, noticing sensations. If images or thoughts come up, notice that, too.

Now invite back the first emotion, noticing if it feels different or the same. Then invite back the opposite emotion. Alternate back and forth between the two, noticing.

Maybe experiment with welcoming both emotions at the same time.

Then let this go and come back to your breath. Repeat again with any sets of emotions that you would like to explore.

I should be grateful

Though the true spirit of yoga involves welcoming ambivalence, an unfortunate tendency in modern yoga is to avoid ambivalence by insisting on only "thinking positively" or "cultivating gratitude." We say things to ourselves like, "I just need to trust the universe," "I'm just going to focus on love," "I am not going to live in a place of fear," or "I just need to decide not to be anxious anymore."

Moms may also fixate on "manifesting" what they want. "I want a beautiful and peaceful birth, so I will just think about that and manifest it;" "I'm sure my baby is just colicky because I am so anxious. If I just manifest being calm myself, my baby will follow." Manifesting is a magical belief that if we just want something badly enough, it will happen.

Some people mistake positive thinking for emotional wisdom, believing it is standard CBT (cognitive behavioral therapy). They might say, "I just need to replace my negative thoughts with positive ones." But this is not what CBT does! In CBT, you first notice and acknowledge depression and anxiety, bringing awareness each day to what negative thoughts emerge. That awareness is often enough to help with difficult thoughts. If not, you can challenge irrational thoughts, finding thoughts that are more truthful and reality-based, even if they aren't "positive." CBT also focuses on choosing new behaviors. It is so much more complex than "being positive."

Cultivating gratitude and setting positive intentions can be meaningful and effective in many circumstances. But when we jump to gratitude and positivity without moving through our more difficult feelings, something is lost.

This jumping past our problems right to positivity can be called a "spiritual bypass." Spiritual bypass means rejecting your darkness, fragility, humanness, and grief. It means thinking that "being spiritual" should take away all your suffering. It might even mean denying that you experience suffering—pain becomes a "sensation," fear becomes a "misconception."

It also makes it your fault then, when you do suffer, when you get sick, when loss comes your way, because you just haven't been spiritual enough. And if you are blessed enough for things to go as you hoped, for you to have the healthy baby or type of birth you wanted, it makes you miss the miracle of it because you think that you made that happen. Spiritual bypass can also make it harder for other people to connect with you because it might make them feel like they can't share their sadness, anger, loss, and pain with you.

Spiritual bypass is another form of attaching to one outcome over another. And it assumes that we get what we deserve. When we face life honestly, without bypassing, we see that, sadly, we often get what we don't deserve. Life has its ups and downs and doesn't always go as we want it to. We all experience loss, sickness, anger, and pain. We make mistakes. We hurt others and get hurt.

Learning to allow the struggles and imperfections of life can give us room to appreciate and make the best of what we have. You may not be able to manifest your baby sleeping through the night, and you may not be able to get the thought *This sucks* out of your mind, but you can enjoy the sweetness of your baby's soft head on your shoulder in the middle of the night, the satisfaction of your deep yawn in the agony of exhaustion, the kindness of your partner as they take over with your baby for an hour so you can nap.

It's not really possible to get through life feeling happy or "spiritual" all the time. When we surrender to our suffering and the suffering of others, when we are willing to welcome it with open arms, we might begin to see that suffering is only one part of the landscape of our wholeness. This is what I mean when I talk about awakening— awakening to compassion, openness, and the vast spaciousness of what it means to be alive.

Practice **Surrender in Savasana**

Savasana, or corpse pose, is often described as "the most difficult yoga pose." While it doesn't require physical strength or flexibility, it does require a willingness to surrender. The name "corpse pose" may sound morbid, but it actually allows us to come face to face with what it means to stop striving, fixing, or manifesting, and just be.

Here are instructions for savasana in pregnancy and postpartum.

Pregnant
Lie down on your side. Knees can both be bent. Alternately, bottom leg can be straight, with top leg bent, with pillows supporting top knee and ankle.

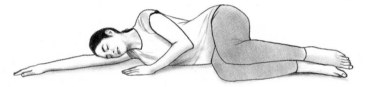

Savasana in pregnancy

If you find yourself uncomfortable, you could try any of these adjustments:
- Put a folded blanket under your head.
- Rest the bottom arm under your head or shift it in front of you.
- Rest the top arm on your belly, or on a pillow in front of you.

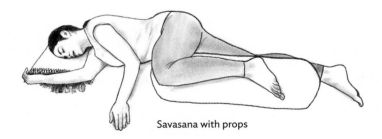

Savasana with props

- Experiment with how many pillows or blankets you might need to support your top leg.
- Shift your hips a little backward or forward to change the curve of the spine.
- Place an eye pillow or arm of a shirt over your eyes.

New moms

Lie down on your back, arms open to your sides, legs straight out.

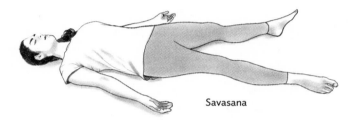

Savasana

If you find yourself uncomfortable, you could try any of these adjustments:
- Put a folded blanket under your head.
- Put a few pillows under your knees.
- Cover yourself with a blanket or sweater (or baby blanket, if that's all that's nearby!) if you are cold.
- Externally rotate your upper arm bones to help your shoulders soften.
- Notice whether it feels good to have your arms open to the side. If not, try resting your hands on your belly.
- Place an eye pillow or arm of a shirt over your eyes.

Once you take your pose, give in. Don't worry about forcing yourself to relax—just let your body be. Let go of any attempt to breathe a certain way or have a clear mind. Let go of being calm, or happy, or good. Let whatever feelings are present—be they rage, grief, sadness, joy, numbness—all come your way. No need to fix, no need to do anything at all.

Uncertainty

When I was about seventeen weeks pregnant with my first child, I told a friend who had two older children all my worries about my baby's health. I said, "I'll stop worrying after the eighteen-week ultrasound, when I see that everything's okay." She laughed. "Oh, honey," she said, "You won't ever know that everything is going to be okay. You won't stop worrying about this kid until the day you die. Welcome to motherhood!" She was right. The uncertainty about what will happen to our children, the wondering if they will be okay never ends.

Learning to tolerate uncertainty, to cultivate *equanimity* in the face of not knowing, is one of the main teachings of yoga—and wow, does parenthood give us plenty of opportunities to practice.

Unfortunately, dealing with uncertainty can be really tough for people with anxiety. Worries flow and compulsive behaviors like planning, checking, researching, and avoiding can give the illusion of control, a defense against the fact that we never really know what will happen to ourselves and our children. Alternately, people with anxiety might struggle to make decisions or even to fully prepare for upcoming events, to avoid the anxiety over whether they might have made the wrong decision or prepared in the wrong way.

We can face this struggle by balancing preparation with acceptance.

We can begin by noticing all the ways we prepare ourselves—the ultrasounds, the birth plan, the "due date," reading books about pregnancy, getting the nursery ready, choosing what kind of bottle nipple or swing or carrier we think our baby might like, learning about parenting skills, and fantasies of the future. We can move forward with these things, in a way that makes sense, creating for ourselves an inner compass. Then we can respond flexibly to the unfolding reality.

A great example of this is the birth plan, which I wish we could rename, the "birth preference list." It's both empowering and practical for your loved ones and providers to know what would feel safe and containing to you. You can list where you want to give birth, who you want in the room, how you want people to talk to you, what interventions you want to avoid, what comfort measures you want to have taken. These decisions are so important as a way of advocating for yourself, and for communicating with others at a time when words may leave you.

Then you let go of that birth plan if you need to. You can absolutely set intentions and invite the optimal circumstances for yourself, but sometimes life comes in with its own plans. I know people who have planned a home birth and ended up having a cesarean birth. I know people who have planned a hospital birth with an epidural and ended up giving birth at home with just their partner present. The births of my two daughters, each begun with the same "plan," were wildly different. The pacing, the pain, and the sensations in my body were completely different each time because my two babies were each in a very different position. It would have made no sense to birth my babies in the same way.

You don't know what day you are going to give birth, how long it will take, what might be easy, what might be hard, where you might find moments of joy or laughter, and where you might have moments of terror or anger. You don't know how you will feel. You don't know what your baby will need. You don't know if you will feel up to hosting friends to come meet the baby in the first week. You don't know what your mood will be like, or how much sleep you will have.

And thank goodness! When we have certainty about how everything will go, we're left with no room to respond to the moment or to try or to discover something new. Embracing uncertainty can allow us to work with whatever comes up.

Note what comes up internally if things don't go the way you hoped. Note how you might judge yourself, get angry at others, or feel betrayed by your faith or your body. Welcome these thoughts and feelings, offering yourself compassion—it's so painful when things do not go as planned. And then you can experiment with adding in new thoughts. You can tell yourself, "I will work with whatever happens, I can be flexible, I am not in this on my own. Every living being on this earth is here with me, facing uncertainty."

Practice **Wave Squats**

I learned wave squats from my teacher, Jane Austin, and for me they were the perfect yoga asana metaphor for developing equanimity in pregnancy. Jane teaches them in every prenatal class and extolls the benefits of doing them for keeping a healthy pelvic floor in pregnancy and beyond. I love how they stretch and activate every part of my body, from my arms and legs to my back and hips. I love how they make me feel fluid, rhythmic, flexible, and strong. I love going through the parts of the movement that feel like intense work and greeting the parts that feel like sweet release. I cultivate equanimity by keeping a constant breath throughout changing cycles, truly embodying "going with the flow."

- Start with feet about a mat's distance apart, toes pointed forward.
- If squatting isn't something you do every day, fold up a blanket or towel and put it under your heels to give yourself an extra inch of height.
- Bring the hands together at the center of the chest.
- Inhale and squat down as far as is comfortable, with the seat coming no farther down than the knees.
- Exhale and tip yourself forward, releasing the head and arms as you straighten your legs, coming into a standing forward fold with knees slightly bent.

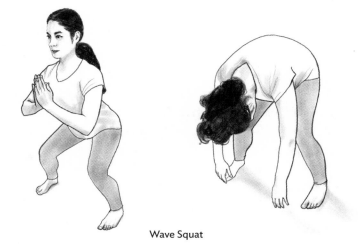

Wave Squat

- Roll yourself up slowly, keeping knees bent and face, arms, and buttocks soft. As the head comes up, arms reach up to the sky.
- Palms meet one another and then, as your inhale begins, draw palms back down, past the head, to return to the center of the chest. Lower into your squat again.
- Continue this movement several times, allowing it to become seamless and fluid, linked with each breath. And if it makes you feel dizzy or nauseated—choose another practice.

The darkest thoughts of depression

Many moms suffering from PMADs experience thoughts about death. It can be scary to acknowledge the darkest thoughts that you may experience when you are depressed. We may fear that talking about them will give us more thoughts, or, worse, make us more likely to act on them. We may fear that talking about them will let others know how bad and crazy we really are or may lead to someone trying to take our baby away from us.

If you have thoughts like this, you don't have to push them away or tell yourself that you are not "supposed" to have them. To heal, it helps to share, out loud, that those thoughts are there and listen to what is underneath them. Talking about suicidal thoughts actually brings them to the light. In yoga, the quality of light, or *sattva*, invites truth, wisdom, and clarity. Facing our thoughts enhances our ability to welcome each aspect of our experience. It helps us figure out what we need and what to do. It helps us feel truly heard.

In the spirit of bringing all thoughts out of the shadows, here are some thoughts you may find yourself encountering:

- This would all be easier if I just weren't here.
- My baby or family would be better off without me.
- If I were to die it would be a relief.
- I wish I could kill myself but I wouldn't do that to my family.
- I wish I could kill myself but I'm too tired.
- What a terrible person I am for even thinking this—I really deserve to die.
- I'm afraid I might actually kill myself. I can't stop thinking about it.
- I want to kill myself. I'm researching options.

In yoga therapy, we look beneath these thoughts to what they are truly mean to express. What are your thoughts pointing to? What are they telling you about your soul or your body? For most people, thoughts of suicide and death can be translated to mean:

I feel distress, and
I need an escape, or
I need relief.

Sometimes it works better to say these things, clearly, to yourself and to people in your life, than it would to just share the original thoughts on their own. It can be easier to come up with solutions this way.

Talk to your support network and get them in there to help you. Ask, "How can I get some relief? How can I get an escape?" Maybe they can help create a plan for more breaks, more sharing of responsibility, more childcare, more time off from working.

Let me be very clear here: If you are having serious suicidal thoughts, yoga is not going to be enough. Don't be alone. You need support. You will need professional help from a licensed mental health professional, and as soon as possible. You may also need or want to spend time in a hospital or outpatient program until you feel safer. That's okay, too.

And if you have to wait a few hours or days to get professional help, many moms find support by calling a hotline or warmline. The National Suicide Prevention Lifeline has a hotline at 1-800-273-8255. Postpartum Support International has a warmline just for moms with these thoughts and feelings: 1-800-944-4773.

Practice **Yoga Therapy Distress Tolerance Tools**

If you are worried that you might actually harm yourself or someone else, please tell a loved one, go to your nearest emergency room, call a hotline, or reach out to your care providers. If you know you are safe, but just need to survive a wave of the darkest thoughts, here are four strategies:

1. Move If you have a thought like, I just need to DO SOMETHING right now to feel better, try some of the dynamic practices on page 109 on moving with anxiety. Walking vigorously can help, too.

2. Take a break If you are wishing for an escape, take a real break. This will mean asking someone else to care for your baby. Find a place that is quiet or put on some music that feels soothing. Get in a resting pose like savasana (page 128). Be sure to make it comfortable with pillows and blankets. Stay there until you have had enough. If you don't feel up for turning inward, you could watch a movie.

3. Use kind and compassionate self-talk Offer hope and patience to yourself. You might tell yourself things like: "These are really hard thoughts to have," "Thoughts are human," "Thoughts come and go," "Thoughts don't mean I will act on them," "This baby will not be a baby forever," "You will feel better in time, "People recover from depression."

4. Ride the wave of feelings Ask yourself what you are feeling. Label it. Then sit and watch the feeling for some time; see how it rises and falls in intensity; learn the pattern of the waves, how big they get, what happens at their strongest, and what it is like as they wane.

My baby won't stop crying

There will be times when your baby will not stop crying. You may be in the car, unable to soothe them as they wail in the back seat. You may be at home, in the middle of the night, and your baby has colic or is teething. Maybe you are out in public, and you think others are staring at you, thinking you are not a good parent.

You might run yourself ragged—feeding, changing, bouncing, shushing, singing, beating yourself up for all the ways in which the baby being unhappy is your fault ("I should have put her down earlier"; "It's because I ate broccoli"; "It's because I was anxious when I was pregnant") or worrying about what it means for the future ("She'll always be an unhappy person"; "This is a sign something is seriously wrong with her").

When you notice these thoughts, you can slow down and tell yourself that you have an opportunity to let your baby know that all feelings are welcome, none last forever, and they do not need to be silenced. You love them and can be present with them even if they are in distress—especially when they are in distress. Don't you wish someone would say that to you?

Babies are people, just like you. They have intense feelings. It's okay, even healthy, for them to express and vent these feelings.

You can't always get it right or anticipate your baby's every need. You can't read their mind. There is no such thing as a perfect mother who meets her baby's needs so completely that they don't ever cry.

You might try riding the wave of your child's feeling. This means holding and maybe rocking your baby without trying too hard to quiet them. Their cries might get more intense before slowing down. You can say to yourself, "I can tolerate this." Of course, tolerating loud cries is hard because your nervous system is cued to react strongly to the sound of your child crying. You will need to practice letting go of the urge to quiet them, offering just attention and love. Don't do too much. Sit with them. Look at them. Soften your own body and practice being receptive.

I know it may sound silly, but it can be helpful to speak aloud to them, especially if you are in the car and cannot physically offer connection or comfort. You might say, "You are so upset. I really hear you. Thank you for telling me how you feel. I'm here to listen. You can cry as long as you need to. I'm right here. I'm with you. I love you." Practice saying this calmly and softly, letting go of any attachment to making the crying stop. While they won't literally understand your words until they are a little older, they will feel your ease and caring. A calm voice soothes both of your nervous systems and the words may help you feel like the mom you want to be.

This is great practice for what's ahead. Because while your baby won't understand what you say to them right now, your toddler will, your teenager will, your someday-adult child will. I have found this approach has saved me many times from yelling at my kids and feeling guilty afterward.

Once, my daughters were given plastic rings as goody-bag presents. My five-year-old got a pink ring, and my two-year-old got a purple ring. The five-year-old, exhausted from a busy and exciting party, saw that she didn't get the purple ring and felt upset. She asked her sister to trade. Her sister said no. The five-year-old started to whine unreasonably loudly. When this didn't work, she began to cry hard, wails coming out of her mouth, snot dripping from her nose.

Everything in me wanted to say, "Everyone gets what they get. It's just a plastic ring. Stop being so difficult and stop crying!" Instead, I took a deep breath and tried, "I know, I was an older sister, and I always felt jealous when my little sister got things I wanted. You are so disappointed. I'm sorry. It's hard when you don't get what you want." She hugged me, and I let her snot rub into my shirt. I let her cries into my ears. Her crying started to slow. I am surprised to find, each time I do this, that not only does the crying cease more quickly, but my love is greater, too. I end up seeing her in deeper color. Sometimes all our children need is to be seen.

As a therapist, I see well-intentioned, loving parents who struggle to tolerate seeing their child or teen suffering without trying to fix it. Instead of saying, "You are so upset. I really hear you. Thank you for telling me how you feel. I'm here to listen. You can cry as long as you need to. I'm right here. I'm with you. I love you," they say, "You wouldn't be so upset if you had just done your homework earlier," or "if you had different friends," or "if you just. . . . " Then the child or teen, feeling shut down, no longer wants to share painful feelings with the parent, leaving the parent feeling like a failure. If we stop measuring success by the absence of difficult feelings, we might feel like successful parents more often!

Practice **Compassion for Baby**

Say to your crying child, "You are so upset. I really hear you. Thank you for telling me how you feel. I'm here to listen. You can cry as long as you need to. I'm right here. I'm with you. I love you."

My baby has been up for hours, and I can't sit down

In the first few months of your baby's life, you will find yourself needing to walk back and forth with your baby, bouncing, *shhhh*ing, giving constant motion to simulate what it was like for your baby in your womb. This walking can sometimes feel sweet, an opportunity to care for and connect with your child. It can, however, sometimes feel like torture, especially if it is in the middle of the night.

Many moms describe a train of thought like, *I just can't do this anymore. Am I a bad mother for wanting some sleep? Will my baby be messed up because his mother didn't want to walk him back and forth? I need to sit down. Please, please fall asleep, baby!*

I first thought of the title of this book at just such a moment, when my second daughter was six months old. I made a hormonal and questionable choice to take her with me to an overnight mindfulness retreat. I had dreamy images of myself as a mindful mom in a stock photo—nursing my baby on a meditation cushion in the glow of the sun, an expression of bliss on my face, a clear mind, surrounded in quiet.

The day we arrived, my daughter started to sniffle and came down with a cold. She was, understandably, very cranky. While everyone else meditated, I had to walk her around and around the back of the room to keep her from crying. My mind fixated on how this wasn't going the way I wanted, how it just wasn't fair! My mind can be really creative—I found reasons to criticize myself for being a bad, selfish mother for going to the retreat. I was angry because no one was saving me. I was angry at my daughter. And I was worried about her—what if this wasn't a cold and was actually a sign that she was very sick? Or going to die?

This went on all day and into the first night, when I had the horrifying realization that since we were at a quiet retreat center all in the same building, every single person there would be kept awake by her howling. And howl she did—every time I tried to put her down. I walked and walked, trying to soothe her. Once I brought her into bed to nurse, and she drifted off! Then I moved to keep my arm from falling asleep, the movement woke her, and we were up walking again.

I noticed myself thinking, *I can't take this anymore.* Then, *I'm going to die. This is going to kill me.* After a few very dark minutes, I had the thought, *Hmmm. I haven't died yet.* I laughed out loud. This was just me practicing, observing all of these intense thoughts and feelings. That's when it occurred to me that I could use the mindfulness practice we'd been learning that day, walking meditation, in real life—to become "awake at 3 a.m.," to move with my exhaustion, desperation, and awareness.

Reframing walking with baby as walking meditation can be both a coping skill and an opportunity. It elevates the soothing of your baby into a spiritual practice, which can feel empowering and hopeful. It can also help you hold your resentful thoughts in a different way—not as something to be judged or removed, but something to notice—and to find spaciousness and compassion around them.

Practice **Walking Meditation**

You can walk inside or outside, with baby in your arms, or perhaps in a carrier or woven wrap. Find enough room to walk a path of at least ten steps. It can be nice to practice walking meditation with your shoes off. The tactile experience of feeling your soles on ground can deepen your focus. Without shoes, your feet also have more room to articulate as they move. If you can't take off your shoes, that's fine. You can still feel into the sensation of your feet in your shoes, the press of your socks into your soles.

Start by standing in one place. You may like to close your eyes for a few moments to connect with yourself.

Begin walking slowly down your path, drawing your attention to the sensations in your feet as they move. Notice:

- The slow shift of your weight onto the right foot
- The sensation of weight and balance on the right foot
- The lift of the left foot
- The placing of left foot
- The shifting of the weight back onto the left foot, and slowly off of the right foot
- And so on

When you reach the end of your path, turn around, and continue in the other direction. You may notice the mechanics of your feet as they help you turn. When your mind wanders, gently and calmly bring your attention back to sensations in your feet, over and over again.

Some people find it helps them stay steady in their attention if they use words to name each movement. You might think to yourself: shift, lift, place, shift, lift, place.

If you are walking with baby, and they keep crying or—maddeningly—fall asleep and then cry whenever you stop moving, notice the reactions that come up. Do you have thoughts like *Stop crying!* or *I need this to end!* When these exhausted or frustrated thoughts enter your mind, you can practice self-compassion. Tell yourself that it is a reasonable and normal human response to wish your baby had a pause button and you could take a nap. You can also practice compassion for baby (page 139) or gently bring your attention back to your feet. Keep walking.

When you have finished walking, take a moment again to stand on both feet and notice the effects of your practice.

Grief

Grief is not a feeling that many would associate with pregnancy or new motherhood, yet this time of many blessings is also one that can bring the greatest losses. Many parents have experienced some kind of loss, perhaps a miscarriage, an abortion, a stillbirth, or the loss of a child. Grief can also be related to the loss of experiences. For example, if a baby has health problems that lead to a stay in the NICU, or has ongoing special needs, parents must grieve the experience they had envisioned having, or the child they had dreamed of.

Grief is a normal reaction to loss. It comes in waves, feelings of sadness, anger, fear, and disbelief, rising and falling. Sometimes we feel nothing—just numbness. Other times, it feels as if it will never end. Grief also tends to come on strong on anniversaries—days that remind us of the loss we suffered or make us wonder what our lives would have been like if our loss hadn't happened. In pregnancy and new parenthood, with so much focus on weeks, months, milestones, and birthdays, the waves of anniversary grief can feel unrelenting.

Depression turns these waves into tsunamis, blowing toward us and those we love. You may judge yourself for not "getting over it" more quickly. You may tell yourself that you caused your loss, that if you had just done better, you could have prevented it. You may be angry at others who haven't suffered such a loss, because it's just not fair. You may be angry about things people have said to you that feel callous, ignorant, or lacking in compassion.

Anxiety, too, makes the waves treacherous. You may perseverate on what you could have done differently, and fear that you could experience loss again. You may have a very hard time feeling safe, or allowing yourself to feel joy, for fear that you will have to feel sadness again.

Grief has no timeline for healing, and the best medicine is compassion: making space for all the painful feelings, and offering ourselves understanding and love. This can be tough. Most of us humans have a strong urge to reject painful feelings, to turn away from them. The root of the word *depression* is *press*—we press away, press down our pain. Yoga, instead, offers the opportunity to lift up our pain, to find space around it.

Practice **Welcoming Suffering/Offering Compassion**

Karuna is the Sanskrit word for compassion. "Welcoming suffering" is a form of karuna, a compassion meditation in which we purposefully make space around painful feelings. The Buddhist name for a similar practice is Tonglen.

To practice compassion, we turn toward our suffering, not only letting it be, but also kindly inviting it in. Sit in meditation and say these words to yourself as you breathe:

As I inhale, I welcome and breathe in my suffering.

As I exhale, I breathe out kindness and understanding.

We can also practice this in a more inclusive way, welcoming not only our own suffering but the suffering of others. In this way, we let our suffering be a source of connection rather than separation. We might say to ourselves:

As I inhale, I welcome and breathe in my suffering and the suffering of others.

As I exhale, I breathe out kindness and understanding for myself and others.

This type of meditation is often practiced as a way to be with the suffering of others, such as those who are sick, lonely, or dying. You might try offering it to your baby when they're crying, or to your partner who is just as exhausted as you, or to your older child who is struggling with this new baby. You might offer it to all the other moms out there, bouncing their babies, wishing for sleep, gazing out at the moon at 3 a.m.

It's important to note that this practice does not mean we are transforming a negative emotion into a positive one. The wish of lovingkindness isn't meant as a release of suffering, or exhaling out the bad stuff. Instead, we absorb the suffering. We show ourselves, I am spacious enough to contain even this. We view lovingkindness as a breath of air that gives us the courage we need to return to face the suffering, again and again.

Welcoming suffering can be especially helpful at times where you don't want to be positive, nice, or happy, when depression feels thick and demanding. Sometimes, however, the pain is too much for a welcoming meditation to feel safe. It may feel like the pain would just knock you over. That's okay. You might try focusing instead on simply sending out wishes of kindness and understanding to yourself and/or others.

Section Three
Cultivate Self-Compassion and
Let Go of Comparisons

The pressure to be a "good mother" can feel overwhelming. In a world where moms are expected to meet their child's every need while also making organic food, cleaning the house, looking "together," and succeeding at work, it's easy to get caught in painful comparisons and perfectionism. In this section, you will cultivate self-compassion and learn yoga therapy tools to help let go of judgments, insecurities, expectations, and "shoulds," allowing yourself to just be a human being.

This is hard

Pregnancy is hard. Having a baby is hard. Having anxiety or depression is really hard. And yet, it's so challenging for many moms to acknowledge this for ourselves. We do everything we can to reject our own suffering.

Moms say things like:

"It's not really a big deal."

"It's easier for everyone else. If it's hard there must be something wrong with me."

"It's not like I have cancer or anything."

Most of us have heard the golden rule, "Do unto others what you would have them do unto you." While this is a crucial message for our society as a whole, it makes an assumption that may not be true— that we would automatically treat ourselves better than we would treat others.

So many new moms treat others better than we treat ourselves. We feed our babies at the first sign of hunger, while ignoring our own needs. We lovingly bathe our babies and moisturize their bodies after each bath—but when was the last time we sweetly moisturized ourselves? When our children fall and hurt themselves, we hold them and say, "Oh, honey, ouch! That must have hurt." But when was the last time we said to ourselves, "Oh, honey, this is a big deal—this hurts"?

The word *compassion*, or *karuna* in Sanskrit, means to be with the suffering of others—to feel their suffering, care for their suffering, and connect in a spirit of shared humanity. When feeling compassion, we put ourselves in another's shoes and know that their suffering makes sense in the context of their lives. We offer them love and wishes of ease and healing. Self-compassion turns that understanding and care toward ourselves.

With self-compassion, we remind ourselves that we are human and fallible, and connected to all other human beings. We acknowledge our suffering and extend the balm of lovingkindness to ourselves. Happily, this often makes it possible for us to follow the golden rule—we will often be so much better able to love others if we feel internally grounded. What a powerful tool for us as mothers who so hope to have our babies feel loved.

When I talk about self-compassion with my clients, they often roll their eyes at me. They worry that if they acknowledge their own pain, they will drown in it. They worry it will make them self-pitying, weak, self-indulgent.

Once I was in the grocery store with my daughter, and she was crying because she wanted to buy some candy at register, and I wouldn't let her. She buried her face in my leg, and I said, soothingly, "I know, baby, life is hard." A man nearby looked at me angrily, and turned to her and said, "Don't listen to your mom—life is wonderful!" When I got over feeling stunned and a bit embarrassed by his words, I began to wonder: why is it so scary to admit that life is hard? Life *is* hard—it contains much suffering. And why does acknowledging that life is hard mean that life isn't also wonderful?

I think we all have a bit of this man within us, afraid that acknowledging suffering means we are being negative, or shutting out happiness. But what he missed is that my daughter felt deeply accepted by my acknowledging her struggle in the moment. She started to calm down, and we were able to have a nice talk about how to deal with not getting what we want.

Self-compassion works like this. When we practice self-compassion, our suffering is seen and heard. We don't drown in darkness, weakness, or self-pity. Instead, from a place of acceptance, we find our strength and we are able to feel connected to others. Talking to ourselves with self-compassion makes us more productive, better partners, kinder to others, and, more importantly, less miserable.

Practice **Self-Compassionate Statements**

When you feel intense suffering—sadness, anger, depression—try saying to yourself in a very kind voice:

> *You are suffering.*
> *It's understandable that you feel this way—this is hard.*
> *You are doing the best you can right now.*
> *You are allowed to be human.*
> *I am so sorry this feels so awful.*
> *You need a lot of love around this.*
> *I really hope this gets easier.*

Practice **Self-Massage**

One way of treating yourself with kindness when you're suffering is to give yourself a massage. Yoga self-massage is highly recommended for depression and body image struggles, as well as post-childbirth. You do not need any oil, but if you have a few minutes to do this with oil, it can often feel like a real treat.

You might find it's easiest to do after a shower, still in the shower, with the water turned off, so you can turn the water back on and rinse off afterward. You can use any oil in your house—coconut oil, olive oil, almond oil, sesame oil. I like coconut because it smells good—it reminds me of the beach! It can be nice to warm the oil by putting the bottle or jar into a bowl of hot water for a few minutes (or keeping it in the shower with you).

You can massage yourself any way that you like, but try to include your scalp, ears, arms, belly, and legs. Breathe easily and bring mindful awareness to the massage, increasing awareness of a pleasurable moment.

Here are some massage gestures you could try:

- Rub palms together till they are warm and then place them on your eyes for three deep breaths.
- Make circles all around your face and jaw.
- Use fingers and fingernails on your scalp.
- Massage the back of your neck and top of your shoulders.
- Lift each arm in the air. Using the opposite hand, grasp the upper arm right by the armpit. Slowly and firmly run the hand all the way up to the wrist.
- Massage the hands, squeezing and pulling on each finger.
- Make circles around your heart and chest with both hands.
- On your belly, make big clockwise circles.
- Rub your lower back with your thumbs.
- Slide your hands down each leg.
- Massage the feet, squeezing and pulling on each toe.

If you have your baby nearby, they may really enjoy an oil massage, too—not to mention your partner! Giving one another oil massages can be a beautiful way to connect.

How will I get through the rest of the day?

Sometimes I get a call from a client who is desperate and tearful. "How will I get through the rest of the day?" she asks me. She's tried everything we've worked on, and it isn't enough—it's really bad. She's overwhelmed. She's exhausted. She's been up since 5 a.m. The baby won't stop crying, or climbing, or pulling things off of shelves.

She's full of dread for the hours ahead.

We make a plan: when can you next get some childcare, when does your partner come home, who can you call for help, when can you see your doctor, when does your support group meet, when is your next yoga class? But then after we make the plan, there comes the question again: "But how will I get through the rest of the day? What can I do right now until help comes?"

In these moments, it's really important to remember that it's okay to do what you need to do to get through. It's okay. It's just okay. You don't have to make a nice dinner, you don't have to clean the house, you don't have to do that work project you promised yourself you'd finish this week. You don't have to respond to your friend's email or wear something that looks cute. You don't have to shower. You don't have to practice yoga.

Sometimes self-compassion means you are just going to do the nicest thing for yourself right now. You are going to do what gets you through until your break or your support arrives. As long as it's safe, it's okay to do what you need to do right now.

Sometimes moms in therapy say they really need me to give them permission because they just can't give it to themselves. It's even hard for them to say that they want help when a partner offers it. The partner might say, "Do you need me to take the afternoon off to help you?"

And they just don't feel that they can say yes. They think it makes them seem crazy, weak, burdensome, or self-indulgent.

So, in hope that it works, I am going to give you permission right here:

It's okay.

It's okay to stop.

It's okay to put the TV on for a while—to watch it yourself or with your baby.

It's okay to watch something you think is stupid or trashy.

It's okay to go for a walk in your pajamas.

It's okay to cry really loudly and have snot all over your face.

It's okay to hire a sitter or ask your partner or friend to leave work and come babysit for a while so you can go to Target and roam the aisles aimlessly, or go to a movie, or take a nap.

It's okay to tell your friend or partner or even your baby how hard a day you are having and how you can't wait till they are older and don't wear diapers.

It's okay to eat ice cream.

It's okay to hang with your baby—to give up for today on keeping them on a schedule, going to a class, or putting them down for a nap. Just do what freaking works.

It's okay to put the baby in the car and drive around in circles for two hours listening to music or podcasts.

It's okay to call a hotline number.

It's okay to complain a lot.

It's okay to ignore everything in this book and not feel your feelings at all.

It's okay.

These things are sometimes called "radical self-care" because they get to the root of what self-care is. They aren't a massage or a pedicure or a bubble bath (though those things are great). They aren't your first choice or what you think you "should do." They are radically boring and radically real.

The truth is our souls are really good at getting what they need eventually. If we need a break and don't allow ourselves one, an even more desperate part of ourselves will likely come forward. We'll take that break by drinking, using drugs, overeating, overexercising, hurting ourselves, or lashing out at loved ones. If we don't want to do these things, we have to make room to really hear our own needs before it gets to that point.

Yoga helps cultivate your ability to see reality, let go of who you think you are supposed to be, and just be who you really are. And maybe the reality of the moment is that being peaceful or mindful, or pulling yourself up by your bootstraps, is not happening. You see your own suffering, let go of judgment, and respond with true loving-kindness. You won't be in this state forever, and this won't always be what you need.

Practice **It's Okay**

Ask yourself: What do you need or want to do right now? What sounds soothing or fun or like a relief?

Figure out how you can get it.

Tell yourself, "It's okay."

Compare and despair

Comparison is a natural and useful tendency of the mind, allowing us to categorize, evaluate, be inspired by others, and "fit in" with others. In the perinatal time period, it helps give us a sense of security when everything seems so confusing. Comparing can help us decide how we want to parent. It may help us feel connected to others. It can also get out of control.

We compare signs of pregnancy—weight gain, belly size and shape, nausea, cravings, aches and pains. When baby comes, comparisons continue. Is my baby growing as fast as hers? Is my baby too small? Too big? She's back to wearing her pre-pregnancy clothes already—does this mean I'm a slob? I look all put together and she doesn't—does this mean I'm selfish or vain? We compare birth stories, baby's sleep, decisions about going back to work. We compare our current pregnancy to our last, one child to another.

PMADs can turn these normal touchstones into something pernicious. With PMADs, these comparisons distort your perception of reality and somehow always point to you or your baby not being good enough.

In Mom & Baby yoga classes, moms flow in and out of practicing yoga poses and attending to their baby. Some days, the baby lies happily on the blanket, cooing and giggling like a baby in a diaper commercial, while mom gets to "do" lots of yoga. Some days, the baby cries a lot, and the mom spends most of the class comforting and soothing.

My first baby was very happy as long as she was held. She's still like that—a very physically connected and affectionate person. When I attended Mom & Baby classes, she would cry as soon as I put her down on the mat. When my daughter cried, I was convinced all the other mothers in the room were annoyed. My mind exaggerated, telling me my daughter was the only baby in the room of thirty babies that cried that much. My mind created a story about this. For the next two years, I would talk about those classes like this: "Mom & Baby yoga was so hard for us. My baby cried so much more than all the other babies—she just wasn't into it."

When I started teaching Mom & Baby yoga a few years later, I was shocked to notice that almost all the babies cried as much as mine had. My story that my baby had been especially loud was not true. I had to laugh and wonder how I had, in my comparing stupor, forgotten this great truth: all babies cry.

I watch this same saga play out when I teach Mom & Baby classes. Inevitably, there are one or two moms who apologize at the end of class for their baby crying. But these moms' babies had not cried any more than other babies! They just had the comparison monster in their minds, saying all the other mothers had it easier or were doing a better job. In contrast, there were sometimes moms whose babies *did* cry the whole time, yet they said "I was just glad to be here with all the other moms and babies, focusing on my breath!" It amazes me how much power the comparing mind has to create totally different interpretations of the very same situation.

Letting go of comparing starts with noticing. It can help to note in your mind, *Aha! I'm comparing,* or *I'm comparing and despairing!* Look for these clues:

- Thinking you or your baby are so much worse than others
- Concerns about size, weight, timing, development (yours or baby's)
- Comparing how you feel inside to how you see all the other moms look on the outside: "I feel like such a slob and she looks so put-together."

Yoga asana practice is a gift to those of us working on our tendency to compare. Most people think of "advanced yoga" as the one that looks the most acrobatically impressive. So it is inevitable that you will compare yourself to an Instagram yogi, to the person next to you in class, or to something you used to be able to do before you were pregnant.

Treat yoga comparisons as an opportunity to really get to know how your human mind works. Each time you notice yourself comparing, you can say to yourself, "Aha! I noticed. Good job to myself for noticing!"

Practice **Yoga Sutra Study**

Patanjali's Yoga Sutras, Sutra 1.33, advises: "By cultivating attitudes of friendliness toward the happy, compassion for the unhappy, delight in the virtuous, and disregard toward the wicked, the mind-stuff retains its undisturbed calmness."[12]

How can you bring this suggestion into your life?

How might this help you respond when:

- Another mom says she is getting plenty of sleep
- You see a mom who is back to her pre-pregnancy weight right away
- You see another baby who seems happy all the time
- A friend is suffering because of trouble nursing and you think she's doing something wrong that's causing it
- Someone says something hurtful or offensive to you

Automatic negative thoughts

Depression is marked by what we, in psychology, call *automatic negative thoughts*. The thoughts might be insults like *I'm stupid. I'm ugly. I'm a failure. I'm unlovable. I'm a terrible mother. I mess everything up.* They also show up as negative predictions—these are the "never" and "always" thoughts: *I'll never be a good mom. I'll just mess everything up. I'll never get better. I'll always feel this awful.* In contemporary psychology, we see these thoughts not only as a symptom of depression, but also as part of what keeps it going.

Yoga teachings view these thoughts in a similar manner. In yoga, we call automatic negative thoughts *samskaras*, sticky patterns or grooves in our thinking that lead to *avidya*, misunderstanding. Misunderstanding, in this context, means that we confuse what is temporary with what is permanent, we confuse a feeling or experience with who we truly are, or we confuse what harms us with what helps us. For example, we might think that these negative thoughts will somehow help us change for the better. *Avidya* is considered the greatest affliction of the human mind and the root cause of all forms of suffering.

We cannot make these thoughts just go away. It also doesn't work to throw negative thoughts at themselves, as in *I'm so stupid for having these thoughts.*

In the yoga sutras, we are told that applying the tools of yoga, particularly self-study and steady practice, helps bring insight and illumination, dispelling misunderstanding. When we welcome our thoughts by sitting in meditation or nonjudgmentally observing ourselves in a yoga practice, we can begin to notice them and see that, at their essence, they are patterns. Having the thought *I'm ugly* is not a brilliant new insight. It's a pattern, a path you've gone down millions of times before.

I like to think of automatic negative thoughts as being like a playlist on a top 40 radio station, rotating the same "greatest hits" over and over again ad nauseam. You are sick of them, but darn are they catchy! And years later, even if you haven't heard them in a long time, you still know all the words by heart! Observing what thoughts come around most often can help you catch them more often, so you can say, "Ah, there's that *I'm terrible at everything* thought again."

Practice **Mindful Rephrasing**

Words are so powerful. They shape how we feel about things, how we learn, and how we create understanding. So choosing to rephrase our thoughts can often create a big inner shift. Mindful rephrasing involves taking an automatic negative thought and changing the words to create a more truthful, reality-based version. You can think of this as another opportunity to practice *satya*, truthfulness.

You can practice mindful rephrasing informally any time, as you go about your day, or you can do it as a more formal, regular practice.

Notice an automatic negative thought that you have now or that you've had recently. Welcome that thought into your attention, perhaps writing it down or saying it out loud. You might notice how it feels in your body to acknowledge this thought.

Now ask yourself, "How could I rephrase the very same thought in a way that is more truthful and reality-based?" It may take you a few tries. Once you have it, consider writing it down or saying it out loud. You might notice how you feel in your body, or what happens when you take a more realistic view of things.

Examples

Automatic negative thought I am ugly.

Mindful rephrase My hair is messy today and I don't like the clothes that I am wearing. I'm feeling exhausted.

Automatic negative thought I'll never feel better.

Mindful rephrase I feel pretty awful right now, and it's been a few weeks of this. I am having a really hard time. I need lots of patience, perseverance, and support.

Automatic negative thought My whole pregnancy is going to be awful.

Mindful rephrase Right now I am having a strong fear about what the rest of this pregnancy will hold for me.

Note: This exercise is not writing affirmations, insisting on positive thinking, or even positive reframing. The new version might still feel painful—but there is a big difference between, "I am always depressed" and "I feel depressed right now." The latter leaves more room for what the next moment might hold. Mindful rephrasing means being accurate and insightful about what is really happening.

Sometimes, when you try this, the automatic negative thought comes back stronger. This can be a good opportunity to welcome in difficult thoughts, and tell yourself that you don't have to make them go away, even as you cultivate seeing things with clarity. Focus on building up your ability to recognize reality, and let the difficult thoughts come and go.

I'm not a good mom

Many of the automatic negative thoughts of new moms with anxiety and depression boil down to one concern: *I'm not a good mom.* This thought can take many forms: *I'm a terrible mom; I'm a horrible mom; I'm bad at being a mom; My baby hates me; I'm messing up my child; My child deserves better; My partner deserves better; All the other moms are better; All the other moms have it more together than I do; All the other moms are happier.*

Our cultural myth that being a perfect mom is both preferable and possible seeps into most women's lives and creates a sense of striving. When we shoot so high, we often end up in a state of collapse, rejecting any attempt to grow or change. You can see this in the language of the mommy blog culture—we are either the perfect "natural mamas" making fresh, organic, all-natural baby purees and decking out our nurseries in all DIY artwork, or we are "scary mommies" or "bad mommies," empowering ourselves by giving children french fries, making fun of the crafting mamas, and writing about resentment toward our children or partners as though confessing a deep and delicious sin.

Thankfully, there is an option in between "good mom" and a "bad mom:" being a "good-enough" mother. The idea of the good-enough mother comes from D. W. Winnicott, a British psychoanalyst who, in the mid-twentieth century, studied the relationships between mothers and babies. Winnicott believed that a "perfect mother" who met all her child's needs immediately, preventing them from ever struggling, wasn't preferable.

Suffering is part of being human, and babies need moments of not having their needs met in order to see that they are separate from their mothers, that they can survive scary moments, and that their mother will come back again. Having a "perfect mother" doesn't allow the child to learn in this way. And attempting to be a perfect mother can make a mom feel depleted, resentful, and insecure.

A good-enough mother still gives a baby unconditional love and care, providing attention, food, safety, and security. But she sometimes fails. She misunderstands a baby's cues. She arrives to meet the baby's needs a few minutes too late. Then, after she has failed, she engages in repair and reconnection, letting the baby express sadness and rage. She makes space for baby to learn that love can be present even when things aren't perfect.

So consider letting go of the idea of being a perfect mom, and focus instead on being a good-enough mom. Ask yourself: "Am I showing my baby love? Am I making sure my baby is safe and fed? Am I making sure my baby has other people in their life who also provide these things? Am I taking care of myself so I can be more present?" If you are doing this—that's enough. That's so very much.

Practice **Nonjudging**

We don't only judge ourselves as good or bad mothers. Sometimes we judge other mothers. I think of all the things I judged other parents for before I had kids and laugh—because I now do so many of those things. I find that parenting my own kids means eating my words for every time I ever judged another parent.

See if you can cultivate an attitude of nonjudging toward yourself and other parents, reminding yourself that most everyone is doing their best given their own unique circumstances.

When I talk to clients about nonjudging, they often "judge the judging," beating themselves up, saying, "I'm just a judgmental person." This is a redundant statement, since all people are judgmental. It's the human condition.

Nonjudging doesn't mean that you don't ever judge—it means that when your observing mind notices a judgment, you practicing letting go of that judgment, connecting to the fact that you or the person you are judging is just a human being, seeing for just one brief second what it would be like to not need to be an expert. You bring your nonjudging in right alongside your judging.

For example, when you say, "I'm not a good mom," you could practice noticing that thought. You could let go of an urge to list all the reasons you are not a good mom. You could let go of an urge to defend yourself to your mind, proving why you are a good mom. You could come back to the moment, finding your breath, asking yourself what you could do right now to be just good enough.

I can't take any more advice!

You will never again experience a time in your life when so many people have opinions about you and what you should do. When you are pregnant or a new mom, people will tell you what and how to eat, drink, weigh, sleep, and work. They will tell you these things about your baby, too. They will give unsolicited advice about how you should put socks on your baby, or hold your baby differently, or use a different kind of diapers.

When I was out in public with my baby as a newborn, I noticed that if she cried, people would look at her and say, "Oh, are you hungry? Maybe you are cold!" This seemingly benign statement, probably meant to connect with us in some way, always stung deeply—I felt like they were accusing me of failing to provide basic food and warmth to my child.

With PMADs, these comments can really sink in and stick. We might internalize what someone says and begin to criticize ourselves. We might feel angry at them and rehearse over and over what we wish we had retorted.

I wish we could teach the world not to say these kinds of things to moms! But the truth is, what triggers one mama is helpful to another, and vice versa. I've had days when one client with PMADs says, "I was so mad that my husband told me to just not clean my house. Cleaning makes me feel better. Letting it be messy makes it worse." Then my next client says, "My friend told me that it was okay to just not clean my house, and it was a huge sigh of relief. I remembered that I don't have to be perfect." One mom says that being told to put her baby on a sleep schedule saved her, and the next says that anyone who suggests sleep schedules is anal and doesn't know her baby. And she's right (at least about the second part)! They don't.

Yoga therapy teaches us that we can respond by cultivating compassion for ourselves when a comment is triggering. It can be enormously helpful to have compassion for the person who said it, too. Perhaps they didn't mean it the way you heard it. Perhaps what they told you was what helped them in a dark time. Remember that everyone is human, and just doing their best. They are not an authority on you.

Learning how to gracefully move on from annoying advice is important from now on. Because parenting advice isn't going to stop now—it keeps coming as your kids grow. We can work on developing resilience and the ability to "take what you like and leave the rest," as they say in Alcoholics Anonymous. Sometimes, you might take a risk and consider the advice, opening up to looking at things differently. You might choose to follow that advice, or you might decide to follow your inner voice and do what feels right to you. Along the way, you find the path that works for you and your family.

Sometimes, to let go of a trigger, we need to speak up for ourselves. "Letting go" is not just an exercise in our minds. Often, letting go can only follow action. If your doctor talks to you about your pregnancy, for example, in a way that feels disrespectful or hurtful, you can let them know that, and share how you'd like to be talked to. And if they don't listen, it's always okay to get another doctor. If a friend tells you that you should feed your baby a certain way, and that way doesn't feel right for you, it's okay to say so. As mothers seeking support, we may have to search for help, advocate for ourselves with care providers, find our voice, and learn to ask questions in an assertive way that cues people to really listen to us.

Practice **Turning Inward**

"Turning inward" or *pratyahara* in Sanskrit, is one of the most essential yoga practices, considered to be as important as breath control (*pranayama*), movement/poses (*asana*), and meditation (*dharana/dhyana*). When we practice "turning inward," we withdraw our attention from external influences.

Often when people give us advice, we ruminate on it. We go over what they said in our minds and present defensive statements, or beat ourselves up for not having met their standards. When you notice yourself engaged in sticky thoughts or feeling hurt, resentful, or worried about advice you've been given, it's a good time to "turn inward."

Find a time when it makes sense to take a pause, and invite your attention inward. Closing your eyes can help. Notice your body, mind, and heart. Ask yourself if what they said makes sense for you. Ask yourself what you would be feeling if they hadn't said it to you. Ask yourself what you believe to be true. If you don't know what you believe, think of someone who you trust, and think about what they would say. See how that feels.

Practice **Cat/Cow**

Cat/cow is my favorite movement practice for turning inward. It also happens to be a great pose for pregnancy, as it gets the weight of the baby off of your back and pelvis and strengthens the abdominal muscles. It brings mobility to tight places in the spine, and teaches you to link up breath and movement. My advice—which you are encouraged to let go of!—is to do this pose every day, even if it's the only pose you do!

- Come to hands and knees.
- **Cat:** As you exhale, draw the belly button in to round the spine, head and tail curling inward.
- **Cow:** As you inhale, lengthen the spine, letting the crown of the head and the top of the tail lift up.

Practice *pratyahara* by following your own internal rhythm as you move from cat to cow, breathing and moving at your pace.

You also may notice how cat pose can enhance the practice of *pratyahara*, literally turning your gaze inward. See if you can maintain that inward focus as you take cow pose and physically open yourself up again.

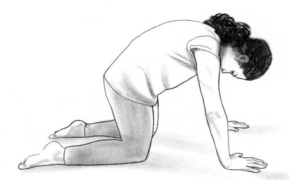

Cat Pose

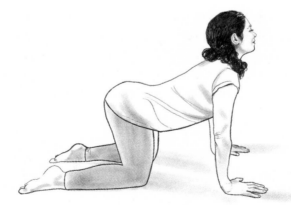

Cow Pose

The all-natural mandate

One of the strange oppressions of modern motherhood is the idea that everything must be "all natural." Doing motherhood in a "natural" way used to mean things like enjoying foods from the earth, or being able to give birth without unwanted medical intervention.

Nowadays, however, "natural" has taken on a moral value, and most moms believe that it means being healthy, virtuous, pure, and good. Choosing things not deemed "natural" is seen as lazy, weak, toxic, and ignorant. This value has become a context for judging ourselves and others (and gives us another reason to be worried about how others will judge us). Many moms feel a need to apologize for anything that doesn't meet this standard, whether it is in the form of medication, an epidural, a bottle, or formula.

These attitudes are especially prevalent in the yoga world. I feel great sadness when I hear about moms going to prenatal yoga and leaving feeling worse about themselves because someone made judgmental comments about something they were planning to do, like giving birth at a hospital, putting their baby in a crib, or heating up their baby's milk in the microwave.

The natural mandate permeates all kinds of everyday decisions. Moms worry about giving a baby some Tylenol for teething pain, or baby food in a jar, or bread. But what does the word "natural" even mean? Who gets to decide what is natural and what isn't? Some foods or supplements that we consider natural are just as processed as medications are. Some things that are natural, like arsenic, can be deadly. Some things that are not natural, like IVF or cesarean births, can create or save precious lives.

The natural mandate is especially painful when it is applied to birth. I often hear the idea that a birth has to be "natural" for a mom to truly experience her power, her spirituality, her womanhood, and her connectedness to her baby. This comes across in sometimes smug celebration of a woman who was "so strong and amazing" for having a natural birth, or in pity of someone who "ended up" with a cesarean birth or epidural.

Yet here is what yoga truly teaches us: a spiritual experience is available in any moment. You don't have to be in pain to have one. You don't have to be in nature, or be doing something "natural" or primal. You can have a spiritual experience in a cesarean birth. You can have a spiritual experience while taking medication. You can have a spiritual experience on the toilet! Yoga teaches us that our true divine nature is always here, accessible and unchanging, not only there under certain circumstances.

Your labor is not your one opportunity in life to truly experience your power, your animal nature, your womanhood, your love. What would that mean for people who don't have children? Or people who adopt? Or fathers? Birth is just one experience—maybe a painful one, maybe a glorious one, maybe both.

The other story I often hear is that natural birth is a feminist experience and that medically assisted births take away women's power. There are some great truths to this—often in medical settings, women experience abuse, fear-mongering, or having their choices taken away. In our culture, profound systemic changes need to be made to respect and support women in labor.

I am a passionate advocate for these changes, and for feminism in general. But frankly, I think it doesn't help the cause of feminism to tell a woman how she should birth, or to say that only a certain kind of birth can be empowering. Only you know what will make you feel empowered and safe. Maybe that's a home birth. Maybe that's a hospital birth. Either way, if you can turn inward, you can see that you are already powerful, and you already contain your wholeness—before, during, and after your birth experience.

This shaming of moms around not being "all natural" is especially painful for those with PMADs. Psychiatric medication is often a crucial part of recovery, yet the shame and stigma around taking it can be staggering. I often hear moms who do take medication apologize for not being stronger or more in love with their kid, as though moral character or love should just spontaneously heal mental illness.

Of course, we do not need to reject everything "natural" along with rejecting the mandate. It doesn't help moms feel less guilty having an epidural if we say that having an unmedicated birth is crazy. It doesn't help a mom who buys baby food pouches if we make fun of moms making their own baby food. Home birth, breastfeeding, making baby food—all these decisions can be profoundly meaningful, beautiful, and healing for the mom who chooses them, as well as for her baby. Every mom deserves support, encouragement, and faith in her choices.

We can use all kinds of tools to care for ourselves and our babies. Taking medication is not at odds with practicing yoga therapy as a way to heal. Having a home birth doesn't mean you can't get support from a doctor.

Practice Noticing Ego

Yoga teaches us that one of the great obstacles to our liberation is *asmita*, an identification with our ego, or a false sense of who we are. We label ourselves as good, bad, better than, worse than. We can find freedom by experimenting with letting go of labels one by one.

Ask yourself these questions: What labels do I use when describing my pregnancy, parenting, and birth choices or experiences? How do these labels define me? How do they connect me to other moms? How do they separate me from other moms? How do I feel if I consider letting go of these labels? Who am I then?

Practice Zooming Meditation

One common symptom of anxiety is a need for things to feel "just right." When you have a birth that doesn't go the way you thought it should, you might become fixated, playing it over in your mind, obsessing on how you or your providers could have done it differently. You may have thoughts like, I'll never be able to get over not giving birth the way I wanted to, or I'll never be able to get rid of this nagging guilt that I have, or I'll never forget the image of.... If you have depression, you may have thoughts about how you are "ruined forever."

When you're stuck in thoughts like these, try the skill of "zooming." For example, zoom your perspective back, and look at your birth story as part of the big picture of your life, including all the meaningful moments both easy and hard from early in your life, from the recent few weeks, and in the coming years. Perhaps imagine the richness of life with your child as they grow up, the ups and downs of the teen years, what it might be like to spend time with them as an adult. Without minimizing or denying your pain right now, you can discover the vast spaciousness around that pain, finding beauty in your experience even if things didn't go "just right."

You can develop the skills of zooming by practicing in meditation, zooming in and out from any thought that crosses your mind.

Visualize your mind as a large, clear sky. Sit and reflect on the blue, the vastness, the spaciousness. If a thought comes up, imagine it as a bird or a cloud that appears in the sky. Take note of it, zoom your attention in close, and acknowledge its presence. Then zoom back out, seeing the thought as just one dot in the larger clear sky. Repeat over and over with each thought that comes.

Body image blues

Nearly every mom I know struggles mightily with her relationship to her body, especially after baby comes. Our society is so fixated on thinness that moms often feel like a failure when we can't get our pre-pregnancy bodies "back." Maybe you've called yourself gross, disgusting, ruined, or out of shape. It's hard to honor the change in your body as a sign that your body did the amazing task of creating a human being.

The body image struggle, for me, is a vulnerable and personal topic. I suffered from an eating disorder for many years in my youth. As I healed in my early twenties, I discovered yoga, which helped me learn to listen to and enjoy my body. My body came to feel like a friend. I treasured it, trusted it, and accepted it.

Then I got pregnant, and months after my daughter was born, I found myself inhabiting a different body—softer, bigger, and rounder. I had a pool of soft, wrinkly skin around my belly button. The skin is papery-thin and a bit glittery from where it mixes with stretch marks. The old thoughts I believed I'd left behind—the self-criticism, the disgust, the longing for a "better" body, and the concern about losing control—all came back.

My yoga practice showed up to help me again. It gave me space to create an inner softness and curiosity about all these painful thoughts and feelings. I was able to understand them as my mind grasping for safety, stable identity, and self-esteem at a time when so much was in flux. Just as parts of my body changed, how was my identity changing? How would I hold parts of my old self as I became a mother? Of course it would make sense for my mind to divert these big unanswerable questions to my old obsessions about my size and appearance.

I realized that I could offer myself compassion. "Of course this is scary," I said to myself. "It takes time to accept that things change. I am leaving the part of life where I am a young maiden, and I am moving into being the strong matriarch, a phase in which my hips are wider, my wrinkles (and opinions!) more pronounced."

For many of us, the only way we have been taught to feel better about our bodies is to take on the project of learning to find ourselves beautiful. "Love your body!" we are told. "Embrace your curves!" And I did this myself; I reminded myself that I had expanded to make another person, that my body had done something beautiful and the changes were beautiful. I worked to appreciate the new lines of my curves and stretch marks.

While these are lovely sentiments, they still imply that liberation comes from beauty. This idea distracts us from discovering our true, unchanging nature, the self that has nothing to do with how we look. So I also took care to remind myself, I am not this body. Nor are these thoughts me. This culture has messages about women's bodies that I do not have to buy into, nor do I have to make them go away. The human mind is a sponge, soaking up messages and values from its surroundings. Yet just as the water soaked up by a sponge is not the truth of what the sponge is, these thoughts were not truly me.

Yoga offers us a deeper form of liberation. It frees us to notice our oldest attachments—to things like our bodies not changing, to living forever, to avoiding pain. We open our eyes and face the truth that we cannot hold fast to any of those things. Everything will change. None of us gets our old body back, even if we don't have kids. This is the one and only body we get—how do we live knowing this is it? What really matters? What do you want it to say on your tombstone: *Here lies someone who lost all her baby weight*?

Practice Meditation on Your Changing Body

Gaze at a spot on your body with wrinkles or stretch marks or new fat, welcoming any thoughts or feelings that arise. Just notice any judgments or stories that may arrive, then gently redirect your attention back to the spot on your body. Notice how what you see, feel, and think may change and change as you look.

Practice Soft-Belly Meditation

Allowing and encouraging the belly to be soft can be scary for some moms but also so sweet. So many pregnant women say the thing they love about being pregnant is that they can just let their bellies be soft. It can feel transgressive, given everything we've been taught as women, and also such a relief. Imagine inviting and encouraging your postpartum self to have a soft belly!

Sit (or lie) and notice the breath rising and falling, with the belly as the point of focus. With each inhale, soften the abdominal muscles. You may tune into the sensations of softening as a point of focus, or maybe repeat the words in your head with each exhale—*soft belly, soft belly, soft belly*. Allow the breath to come and go of its own accord. Receive the breath, don't reach for it. Allow the belly to fill and empty without controlling its shape, size, or length.

Over time in the meditation, you may notice deeper and deeper layers of tension held in the belly. Our bodies often hold this tension as an armor against emotional vulnerability or societal standards of beauty. Exhale and allow the softening, again and again.

For some women, it can feel very scary to feel the belly press against the waistline of their pants. You might try practicing soft-belly meditation wearing stretchy clothes or no clothes at all. You may even start to question our society's choices of clothing—why would we wear clothes that don't allow us to fully inhale? Why do we strive to make ourselves fit our clothes, rather than our clothes fit us?

For those who have experienced trauma, letting the belly be soft may bring up painful thoughts and feelings. You may be flooded with fear, vulnerability, and sorrow. If this comes up, decide what action would be kindest toward yourself. For some, stopping the soft-belly meditation might be the wisest choice. Perhaps doing something active with the body—like a walking meditation (page 141) or the physical chores of your day might feel more grounding. For others, it may feel healing to stay with the challenging feelings, allowing them to rise and fall, committing to softening the belly as all sensations are welcomed.

I need to make sure my baby is happy and healthy

I have often thought that the popular book *The Happiest Baby on the Block* has done more harm than good—just with it's famous title. It's actually a great book, providing lovely and useful tools for soothing your baby, but the title promotes the idea that the happiness of our babies is some kind of competition. When you think about it—does your baby really need to be the happiest baby on the block? Isn't it good enough for your baby to just be happy? Is it okay for your baby to sometimes not be happy? My bet is that most—probably all—of the babies on your block are sometimes happy and sometimes sad, sometimes little angels, and sometimes tantrum-throwing messes.

In our society, we put an incredible emphasis on how we mold our children. We are told to read parenting books, eat organic, emulate French parents, sign our kids up for music classes and gymnastics, give them only wooden toys, avoid screen time, give them time-outs so they feel contained, or don't give them time-outs so they don't feel shamed. We try to be mindful parents. And we tell ourselves that we must do everything we can so that they grow up to be happy, smart, thin, disease-free, and very successful. We blame and shame parents when these things don't come true. We're fixated on "optimizing"— once the language of business, and now the language of parenthood.

In trying to optimize our children, we run the risk of seeing them as products or objects—things we make and then are judged on. This way of thinking forces us into a narcissistic stance in which we find our goodness through them. Or we find ourselves living vicariously through our children, avoiding acceptance of our own life's suffering through fantasy: "If my mom had only meditated when pregnant with me, maybe my life would have been better." This can become the ultimate hubris—the idea that our generation, if we optimize our-selves, can create children that are better than every other generation of human animals that have walked this earth: "If everyone meditated when they were pregnant, the whole world would be full of love. We would have no more racism, intolerance, or war."

What if the goal of loving your child were . . . just that—an act of love, rather than a calculated move to make them a happy person? When we get caught up in the frenzy of trying to parent perfectly, we can forget that our children are not things we produce, but actual people. Our job is to care for them, to be curious about their unique needs and talents, and to love them with all their imperfections and struggles. Isn't this a relief?

In yoga, we practice letting go of striving attitudes. We practice the virtue of *aparigraha*, or non-grasping, to let go of attachments to out-come. We soften our grasping by softening our minds, our bodies, and our expectations. Then, we can practice the virtue of *santosha*, con-tentment, finding ease and love for our children and ourselves, just as we are.

We can explore *aparigraha* and *santosha* in our bodies by taking a passive yoga pose. Most of us yoga practitioners tend to push our-selves, stretching hard, sometimes past our body's natural flexibility, tensing up our shoulders or faces just to get one inch "deeper" into a pose. In a passive pose, we avoid stretching into a pose and allow our bodies to find their own shape, enjoying whatever they give us today.

Practice **Butterfly Pose**

Start with the feet together and the knees apart. Sit up tall. Gently release the effort holding you up and slowly let the spine curve forward. You do not have to stretch forward or have the head come down to a certain place. Allow your torso to fall forward to the exact place where your body feels both safe and open. Hands can rest on your feet or the floor. Don't push—just receive

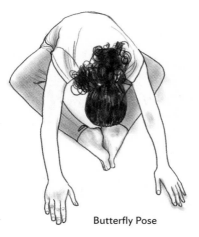

Butterfly Pose

gravity's pull into the pose. Then, stay. Demonstrate acceptance of yourself by finding ease here. Let the awareness settle into a mindful meditation, perhaps with the breath or body sensations as focus. When you are ready to come out, place the hands on the ground, press the arms straight, and very slowly roll the spine upright, bringing the head up last.

Variations
- If your back hurts, sit up on a pillow or folded blanket.
- If your neck hurts:
  - Don't come down as far into the pose.
  - Put a pile of pillows in front of you and rest your elbows on them, then rest your head in your hands. Or
  - Rest your elbows on your shins, then rest your head in your hands.
- If your hips hurt, rest pillows under each knee.
- If you feel pulling or pain in your pubic area, try child's pose instead (page 200).

I often encourage my yoga students, when choosing how "deeply" to move into a pose, to seek out where their edge is and then take a step back from it. Take a shape that allows you to have an even, steady breath.

177

What do they think of me?

Many moms with PMADs find themselves preoccupied with worries about what others think of them. You may worry that they think you look ugly, or messy, or out of shape, that they think your home is a mess, that they think you don't have things together, that you are a bad mother, or that you have become a bad friend. Have you ever ducked out of a family photo because you were worried about what you would look like if someone else saw it?

In psychology, we call this *self-objectification*. Self-objectification is the tendency to view one's life and one's body not as a reality to be experienced, but as an object to be evaluated. When we self-objectify, we are constantly monitoring our outside appearance—how we look or seem to others—instead of focusing on our inner life.[13]

Self-objectification has been linked to increased feelings of shame, decreased attention, disordered eating, depression, and anxiety. During pregnancy, specifically, higher levels of self-objectification have been linked to depression, drug and alcohol use, and lack of self-care measures like adequate sleep, nutrition, vitamin-taking, and exercise[14].

Self-objectification is not vanity or self-obsession—it's something women are taught to do from early childhood. From our first princess movie through adulthood, we are taught that being pretty is what gives us value. We are taught to ask ourselves, "What do others think?" and "How can I make them like me?" when we get dressed, when we speak in class, when we consider careers, and when we look for a date.

Social media amplifies this reality to the nth degree, demanding that we continually objectify our experiences, curating an externally "like"-worthy stream of images that may tell others nothing about our internal experience.

As moms, too, we are taught that self-objectification is a virtue. Typically, from the moment we become pregnant, instead of being encouraged to listen to our hunger and fullness signals to determine how much and what we should be eating, we are directed to a scale, where we get weighed regularly, and are expected to gain a very precise amount each month. If we gain too little—or too much (can't win!)—we are immediately lectured about the danger to our baby. The measures of our goodness and care for our babies become external, rather than internal, right away. We want our babies to be healthy, we want to be good mothers, so we agree to self-objectify. Often, prenatal care doesn't give us opportunities or encouragement to trust ourselves, to believe we can be good mothers to our own babies without someone else's seal of approval.

As you read this, you may notice yourself thinking, *But if I don't weigh myself at my check-ups, I might eat too much! If I don't get measured, I might not exercise enough. What if my baby is too small? Didn't I read somewhere that if a baby is too small it leads to lower IQ and increased risk of depression at age five?* So much pain and fear arise when we think about the risk of letting go of self-objectifying.

The good news is that yoga offers us a way out of self-objectification. Specifically, research has shown that the internal focus of a mindful yoga practice—one that incorporates the tools of body awareness and body responsiveness—significantly reduces self-objectification and its associated ills, including body dissatisfaction and disordered eating.[15]

Practice **Chair Pose from the Inside Out**

In yoga therapy, a key skill we practice is interoception, feeling your body from the inside. Unlike in a regular yoga class, where there is much focus on what a pose looks like, and where you might hear a teacher say something like, "Open the chest. Doesn't that feel good!" or "Press down through the

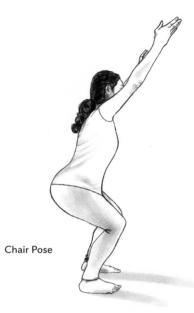

Chair Pose

palms and see how that gives you more stability in your arms," yoga therapy avoids, as much as possible, dictating what a pose should look or feel like.

Here is a guide to practicing interoception in chair pose. You could do this with any pose at all.

Before you take the pose, notice body sensations—pace and depth of your breath, strength, weakness, energy, fatigue, comfort, discomfort, contracting, opening.

Find your way into chair pose, feet a stable distance apart, squatting as though sitting in a chair. Palms can join at the center of the chest or arms could reach up or forward (or be holding a baby!). Get curious about what you feel here, again scanning for body sensations. Notice parts of your body you might usually ignore—what do you feel in your toes? What is happening with your tongue? Your eyeballs? What happens if you sit back a little bit lower? What happens if you bring the weight more into your heels?

As you come out of the pose, notice again. What were the effects of the pose? Scan again for pace and depth of your breath, strength, weakness, energy, fatigue, comfort, discomfort, contracting, opening.

I should...

Often people come into therapy asking me to help them be "better at handling stress." I get very enthusiastic about this because I love to share yoga relaxation skills. But after hearing their story, I realize that it's not that they are not good at handling stress, it's that they have too much stress. There is no yoga practice in the world that can help you relax if you have more responsibilities, more trauma, or more expectations than you can reasonably handle. No yoga and no form of therapy can turn you into a superhuman, able to work twenty-four hours a day. These are the times you need to look at reducing your stress, rather than just "handling it" better.

Often, stress is caused by external pressures—financial, health-related, societal. Other times, stress is caused by what we might call the "shoulds"—all the things we expect of ourselves.

Here are some common shoulds I've heard from the moms I work with, from my friends—and yes, from myself:

- I should be an amazing mom.
- I should respond perfectly to every single cry and coo my daughter makes in order for her to be perfectly attached and therefore have no emotional issues or complexes when she grows up.
- I should lose all my baby weight.
- I should wear real pants every day (no yoga pants, no maternity pants).
- I should practice meditation and yoga for ninety minutes a day.
- I should have breastfeeding down easily and look effortless while doing it in public.
- I should be calm all the time.

- I should have a clean, well-styled house when guests come over to see the baby.
- I should do tummy time with my baby every day.
- I should post more on social media.
- I should go back to work.
- I should stay home with my baby.
- I should have mastered a work/family balance.
- I should be having more sex.
- I should prepare all our food from scratch.
- I should read more.

"Shoulds" don't always come in the form of what we think we should be *doing*. Often they come in the form of how we think we should *be*. We think we should be more grateful, more together, more beautiful, more intelligent, more educated, more caring, more organized. One of the big "shoulds" that I hear a lot, especially from moms who are interested in yoga or mindfulness, is "I should be in the present moment." It always makes me sad when I hear people using yoga as a weapon to criticize themselves!

One of the reasons we think we "should" be in the present moment is that everyone tells us that time with our babies is so precious, it goes by so quickly, they grow up so fast. We may feel guilty about the fact that, perhaps often, this time period feels impossibly long and slow, that we count down the hours till the day ends, and that we wish it would go faster. "What kind of a mother," we ask ourselves, "doesn't want to be in the moment appreciating her baby?" (Answer: lots of them.)

These shoulds come from a good place—a desire to do the right thing, care for our kids, make ourselves feel better. But they also set us up for failure and self-criticism. Because there is no human way to really live up to all our shoulds. We cannot be calm all the time. Our home will never stay clean. We cannot enjoy every moment. We cannot grasp tight enough to appreciating our sweet baby's face that it prevents us from missing it a few months later, feeling that time went by too fast.

Getting lost in these shoulds also prevents us from enjoying things just as they are. If I should be wearing nice clothes all the time, I miss out on enjoying the comfy pants I have on right now. If I should keep my house cleaner, I miss out on how much I love the art on my walls right now when it's messy. If I should make sure not to miss a moment of my kids' precious babyhood, I might miss out on realizing how cool they are as they get bigger.

Practice **Letting Go of Shoulds**

Make a list of your "shoulds." Write down or think of as many as you can.

Look it over, and see if there are any items on the list you wish you could let go of.

Imagine a good friend giving you permission to let it go, saying something firm, like, "Honey—you just do not need to do that. Stop it now. Put the cleaning supplies down. Sit your butt on the couch. It's okay."

Don't reject an idea because it's impractical. Sit with it first. Imagine what it would be like to let that thing go for now. When you imagine, what do you notice in your body? What sensations arise? Where do you clench or tighten? What happens to your breath? What thoughts come up?

Then, consider taking action. Can you let go of a goal of cleaning or returning a phone call? Can you drop the expectation that you will finish everything on your to-do list, or that you will be calm all the time?

The answer will not always be yes. (And don't let this turn into a practice about how you "should" let go of "shoulds"!) But even adding one yes a week can feel truly liberating.

Section Four
Develop Responsiveness and Flexibility

In this section, you will learn about how to take good care of yourself by listening carefully to your body, mind, and heart. You'll learn that you can be flexible in your yoga practice and in your parenting—attending to and choosing what you and your unique family need in each moment to grow and thrive. You will learn how to bring responsiveness to your needs into each moment, to support you in eating, sleeping, feeding your baby, and moving your body with more ease.

But I don't have any time
to take care of myself!

In the midst of all the caring for your baby, it can be easy to forget to take care of yourself. You might feel too tired or believe you don't deserve it—that "self-care" is too self-indulgent.

When we hear the term *self-care*—we picture going to a spa, getting a pedicure, or doing something else we don't have the time or money for. I prefer, instead, using the word *responsiveness* to describe taking care of yourself, listening to what your body, mind, and heart need. Responsiveness means making sure you drink water if you are thirsty, put on a sweater if you are cold, and go to the bathroom if you have to pee.

Don't laugh at that last one. I can't tell you how many moms have told me about how they put off peeing. They are about to pee, then baby cries. They think, *I'll pee as soon as the baby is changed.* Diaper is changed, baby still cries, so they feed the baby. They decide to wait to pee just until the baby is done feeding. Then the baby falls asleep in their arms, and they don't want to wake the baby, so they don't get up to pee. They just sit there, miserable.

It's a good rule that if you have to pee, make that the first priority—just go pee.

Here's a list of basic ways you can practice responsiveness:

- Use the bathroom when you need to.
- Drink water regularly. If you are breastfeeding, try to have water available every time you breastfeed. If you have a partner or a family member helping you, show them this book and tell them I said to bring you a glass of water whenever they see you breastfeeding.

- Eat regularly. Aim for three meals and three snacks per day. Tell that family member to gently remind you to eat and to bring you snacks you can eat with one hand.
- Shower or bathe. When you feel gross, it doesn't help your mood. Feel the warm water on your skin.
- Put on clean clothes, or at least fresh pajamas.
- Get some fresh air and sunshine on your face. Even if it's just opening a window or the front door and standing there in your pajamas.
- Stretch tight parts of your body.
- Stay comfortable: put on something warm if you are cold, take off layers if you are hot, put a pillow behind your back or neck or under your arm when holding the baby for a long time.
- Rest when you are tired. Say no to additional pressures or responsibilities.

Your baby may cry while you do these things. That's okay! Most of these things take less than a minute. Showering takes the longest, and that only needs to be about five minutes. Your baby will be okay if they cry for five minutes—I promise. It won't mess up their attachment to you, and afterward, you will be more available and present.

Yoga is a good playground for practicing responsiveness. Yoga values non-harming, *ahimsa,* so we do not want to hurt ourselves in poses. When people first take a yoga pose, they often focus on what it is supposed to look like, and stay there even if it's uncomfortable, muscles strained and jaw tight.

In savasana, final resting pose, I, like many teachers, often say, "Notice if there is anything your body needs to be even 5 percent more comfortable. If you need any props or any help, let me know." On more than one occasion, a mom has burst into tears when I say this. The idea of doing something to make herself just 5 percent more comfortable is a thought she hasn't had in a long time. Whether she gets a prop for herself or asks me for assistance, she says to herself in that moment, "I hear my body. I care for my body. I matter."

Practice **Responsiveness in Standing Forward Fold**

Start standing on two feet. Traditionally, this pose is taken with feet together—toes touching, heels apart. Not everyone feels steady with feet touching, especially in early pregnancy. Not every body shape makes it comfortable or practical to have feet touch. You may want, instead, to take feet hip-distance apart, toes pointing forward. As your pregnancy continues, you may need to take the feet even farther apart so that you have room for your belly between your legs as you fold. After pregnancy, your body will again be different—you can experiment with the stance that feels right for you each day.

Bend the knees as you fold your torso forward. Let your head be heavy. Let go of the idea of "touching your toes." It might be nice to rest hands on

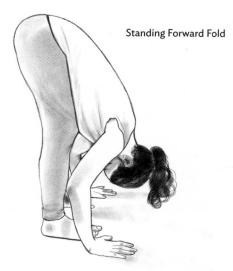

Standing Forward Fold

187

thighs or shins, or blocks in front of you. You might reach around for your calves, so you can use your arm strength to enhance your stretch. It might feel lovely to take hold of opposite elbows, letting the weight of the arms gently traction your spine.

Bring your attention to the lower back. If there is any discomfort at all, perhaps bend the knees further. You could also lift the torso, so you are not reaching so far forward. If your back is comfortable, you may want to experiment with working the legs toward straight.

Last, you can play with bringing your weight forward into your toes and back to your heels. What feels best to you?

When you are done, bend your knees deeply again, bring hands to the thighs, and slowly roll yourself up to standing, head coming up last.

Why didn't anyone tell me?

If I had a dollar for every time a new mom said to me, "No one told me this could happen," I'd be a millionaire ("this" being anything unexpected she might experience in pregnancy or new motherhood). I get it—it is hard to feel caught off guard or not to have a roadmap for what we struggle with. But it is impossible for someone to tell you all the things that may happen in new motherhood. Even if you have been pregnant before, you can't know about all the possible things that can happen. In my first pregnancy, I had upper back pain. In the second, I had pubic symphysis pain. My first child was the greatest sleeper ever (I know—lucky!). My second child still barely slept through the night by three years old.

Maybe someone actually did tell you that some particular thing could happen; you just didn't take it in. I'm sure you've read books or articles or taken a birth class where they listed tons of complications and difficulties in pregnancy, birth, or motherhood. You just cannot keep all possibilities in your head all the time—which is probably our brain's way of helping us avoid living in constant fear. It would take years of schooling on obstetrics, midwifery, pediatrics, and psychology just to understand all the possibilities, much less accept that they could really happen to you. This is like life in general—there is no way someone can list for you all the complications that might happen. Tomorrow you could have an aneurysm, a car accident, an allergy attack, sciatica, a wart on your finger, or a winning lottery ticket.

As often as I hear moms sharing anger about all the things they were not warned about, I also hear moms share anger about all the terrible things people *do* tell them. If someone warns them about pregnancy complications, or the impending lack of sleep, they feel that the person is being negative or pushing fear onto them. This is unfortunate, because that person was probably just sharing the thing that made *them* say, "Why didn't anyone tell me?" in their own pregnancy or postnatal period.

If you hear yourself saying, "Why didn't anyone tell me?" or "Why are they telling me this?!" see if you can let go of focusing on what was or wasn't said, and instead focus on practicing responsiveness to your current situation. This is what is happening now: what is called for now? What do you need?

Responding to and *greeting the present moment* flexibly allows us to take things as they come, and meet whatever is happening to us in pregnancy or parenting, regardless of what others did or did not warn us about. Each day in this time period is an opportunity for great learning and for welcoming in something new. Each day is the first time you have cared for this particular child at this particular age.

Practice Present Moment Focus

We can practice the skill of releasing expectations and greeting the present moment through mindfulness. Mindfulness is defined as the practice of paying attention to the present moment. Our minds travel to the future and the past by nature. I've heard it said that "heart beats, lungs breathe, mind wanders." You are redirecting your very nature when you bring yourself back to the present moment—it's not easy, and it's fairly impossible to just stay there.

Present moment focus is an informal mindfulness practice. You don't need to sit down or set a timer. To practice present moment focus, just right now, in this moment, stop and notice your breath. Notice thoughts, feelings, sensations; notice what you are doing, who is around you, what you see. When your mind wanders, come on back.

Present moment focus isn't choosy. It invites us as we are, with our resentments and our pain. If you are having thoughts about why someone didn't tell you something, or how things are unfair, or worries about the future, notice that, too. You don't have to argue with those thoughts or dispute them. Just notice what is happening right now. What is needed in this moment?

We can pay attention as we are in this moment, letting go of the expectation that we should live in some other, more accomplished body, some more peaceful mind, some braver heart. We can notice what is happening now, what might be "good enough" now, what might even be wonderful now.

We can practice present moment focus at any time—it can work well while changing diapers, burping, feeding, laundering. We can be present with the tasks at hand, knowing they are only for just right now, perhaps finding in them an opportunity to feel that we are doing something sacred.

My body hurts

Having a baby is certainly not ergonomic. In prenatal yoga classes, we start in a circle. Each mom is asked to check in with what kind of support they hope to get out of their yoga practice for today. Though I invite them to share what they might want for their body, mind, and heart, they mostly share about aches and pains in their wrists, back, neck, and feet. They talk about sciatica, pubic symphysis pain, round ligament pain, and carpal tunnel syndrome. Changes in weight, center of gravity, muscle and joint laxity, and—postpartum—the day-to-day physical stressors of carrying a baby everywhere make this a time period when discomfort is almost a norm.

Aches and pains have a circular relationship with anxiety and depression. Having aches and pains can make you feel hopeless, defeated, and stuck, keeping you away from loved activities and leading to depression. Depression can also make you more likely to perseverate on aches and pains, as well as more likely to neglect self-care to deal with them.

With anxiety, perhaps you worry that the pain will never go away, that it will get worse, that you won't be able to function. Maybe you worry the pain means you have some kind of disease. The resulting anxiety creates more pain—if your body is tense, and you are too worried to move your body for fear of making the pain worse, you become more stiff, and more prone to injury.

Addressing aches and pains, thus, is not only an act of responsiveness that helps the body. It also helps with PMADs. When we care for our bodies, we can alleviate some triggers of anxiety and depression. And in doing so, we send ourselves a deeper message, that we are worthy of care, that our pain is seen and heard, that we deserve to be loved.

Yoga therapy teaches us to care for aches and pains three ways:

Self-study Notice and shift daily patterns that cause discomfort. Maybe you sleep in a position that puts too much pressure on your hips. Maybe you cart around a car seat all day, jutting your hip out to the other side as a counterweight. Maybe you forget a pillow for yourself to support your back when you feed your baby. Notice what works and what doesn't work, and come up with small changes you can make to ease the wear and tear on your body.

Find a teacher Yoga philosophy emphasizes the importance of learning from a teacher. A teacher may be able to see things you cannot see, share new ideas, and inspire change. In our modern context, a teacher could be any helping professional who deals with supporting a pregnant or postpartum body. In addition to yoga teachers and yoga therapists, many mamas find relief from working with a physical therapist who specializes in perinatal and/or pelvic floor functionality (especially useful if you have incontinence or pain during sex). Other sources of support include chiropractors, acupuncturists, Pilates teachers, lactation consultants, doulas, massage therapists—the list goes on and on.

Engage in regular responsive asana practice While asanas make great metaphors and help shift the energy in the body, they are also excellent exercises for strengthening, stretching, and stabilizing the muscles to prevent and address aches and pains. You can choose one or two poses to do regularly to address a specific discomfort, or you can create a balanced practice that supports the whole body. A balanced practice would aim for a good blend of poses that strengthen and those that stretch, those that activate the muscles and those that release them.

Generally, a balanced practice includes at least one of each of the following:

A Balanced Asana Practice

1 Standing pose
2 Balancing pose
3 Forward fold
4 Gentle backbend or "heart opener"
5 Gentle twisting pose
6 Restorative or releasing pose

Practice **Flying Cat Pose**

Many aches and pains in the torso come from having instability in the abdominal muscles. Pregnancy is tough on abdominal muscles! If you've had a cesarean birth, you may also experience pain or numbness near your incision. When your abdominal muscles are not working optimally for you, it can become hard to sit up straight. Your shoulders may slump, causing neck and back pain. Even the pelvic floor can be affected by the abdominal muscles, leading to incontinence or painful intercourse.

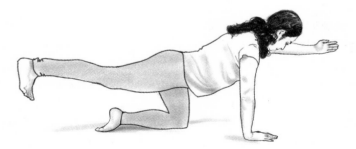

Flying Cat Pose

194

Flying cat pose is a safe and effective pose to strengthen the abdominal muscles during and after pregnancy. It also strengthens the arms, legs, and buttocks, and opens the shoulders.

Come to hands and knees. Find a neutral spine, with a gentle curve at the lower back. Draw the belly button in slightly toward the spine (or toward your baby if you are pregnant). You can also experiment with gently drawing the pelvic floor inward. Straighten one leg out to the back of your mat. You can keep the toes on the floor or lift the leg up to hip height, flexing the foot. Work toward keeping your hips even. You can optionally reach the opposite arm forward, pointing the thumb to the sky to open the shoulder. Work up to staying here for five breaths, and then release back to hands and knees, allowing the abdominal muscles and pelvic floor to soften again. Repeat on the other side.

I'm hunched over all day

When I teach prenatal and Mom & Baby yoga, the most common complaint the mamas come in with is neck and shoulder pain from slouching. Everyone in our culture slouches, especially if we spend a lot of the day reading, typing, or driving. During pregnancy, as we lose connection with our core muscles, our bodies may naturally start to slouch.

After a baby comes, most of us spend a lot of time hunched over our babies, feeding, reading, changing, rocking. We slouch over our babies as we play with them on the floor. Wearing a baby in a carrier can be practical and a wonderful way to bond, but it, too, can pull us into a hunched position. And being hunched over doesn't only hurt our shoulders, it makes it hard to breathe well and can also make us feel depressed, even if we don't have PMADs.

Try it right now as you read. Purposely hunch over and notice what it does to how you feel. You can straighten out again if you like! Now notice what that feels like. For most of us, when hunched over we feel more sad, lonely, uncomfortable, or ashamed; when sitting up we feel more strong, open, and grounded. For some people, however, hunching feels safer and sitting up feels vulnerable or overwhelming. If that's you, then using another tool is okay. Everybody is different.

Renowned yoga teacher B. K. S. Iyengar famously said that open armpits are a cure for depression. When you open your armpits, you broaden your chest. Yoga poses that do so are often called "heart-openers" because of how they make many people feel uplifted. In heart-openers, you have more room in your rib cage to breathe. Your mind notices and responds to the cues that heart-openers send—that you are safe, awake, energized, alive.

While this quick tool may not work when you are in a terribly depressed mood, on some days it will do the trick to help you feel better immediately. Other days, it may give you enough space and energy to notice what you need, get help, or engage in other helpful yoga practices. If practiced regularly, it can be transformational.

Having an open chest takes more effort and awareness to do when core muscles are compromised and weak during or after pregnancy. Give yourself a lot of understanding that it can take time and practice to build up core strength post-pregnancy. There's no need be a perfectionist about sitting up straight all the time. It truly isn't possible to sit up straight all day with a new baby. If you did, you wouldn't get to look at your baby in your arms! Or rest!

Practice Heart-Opening Yoga Pose

There are many yoga poses that can help with opening up your posture. Backbends, side bends, inversions, core strengtheners, and standing poses all fit the bill. Try adding one of the poses or movements below into your asana practice, or even into the middle of your day. You can do all of these while pregnant or with a baby in a carrier.

Easy seated pose Sit with legs crossed. Broaden the collarbones and perhaps imagine a string on top of your head pulling you upright.

Rainbow arms Hold a yoga strap or tie with your hands wide. Keeping the arms straight, lift the strap up overhead as you inhale, bring the strap down behind you as you exhale, lift it back up overhead as you inhale, and then down in front as you exhale. Adjust your hands so you get a satisfying but comfortable stretch. Repeat a few times.

Sun arms Seated or standing, lift arms out to the sides and up as you inhale, palms moving toward meeting at the top, then reverse and bring them back down to your sides as you exhale. Repeat a few times.

Seated or standing basic backbend From either position, lift arms up to the sky and then aim them behind you. Look up toward your hands, keeping the back of the neck long. Perhaps imagine that your breastbone is shooting a ray of light right up to the ceiling.

Seated or standing side stretch Lift the left arm up and reach it over the head to the right. Stay grounded in the left seat, if you are seated, or the left foot if you are standing. Breathe space into the muscles between your ribs. Repeat on the right side.

Standing chest stretch with wall Put your left hand on the wall at shoulder height with your hand wide and fingers pointing left. Turn your body to the right. Keep turning until you feel a nice stretch across your left chest muscles. Repeat on the right side.

Savasana variation (page 128) Lie down with arms crossed overhead and perhaps a pillow under your knees. If pregnant, you can do this while sitting up on a couch or comfy chair and leaning back.

I'm so tired

You feel exhausted. You have thoughts like, *I've never been this tired before*. It takes effort to do anything, and maybe you struggle to find the energy to take care of your baby. You wonder if it's depression, or maybe anemia. You feel desperate for sleep. You try to drown out fatigue with caffeine or busyness, but you end up even more depleted. You think, *What's wrong with me?*

If this is you, you've missed the most obvious reason for exhaustion—that you need more rest. Maybe because your body is building another human, maybe because you haven't had a full night's sleep in months. Maybe because you have deadlines at work, and have to rush to pick up your baby at day care, and the responsibilities never end. It makes sense that you are tired!

Fatigue is the body's way of telling us to slow down. In yoga therapy, we work to help you meet your body's needs for rest. Getting more sleep is a good start, but sometimes sleep may not feel like enough.

Yoga nidra, or "yogic sleep," is a lovely meditation practice that is believed to provide, in one hour, the equivalent of four hours of sleep. You can easily find yoga nidra meditations online (I have a few recordings on my website), or have a yoga therapist make a recording for you.

Yoga asana can help too. At times, you may want to invite in opposite energy—if you've been sedentary for many days and feel stuck, it might be time to get moving. Doing some active poses or sun salutations, in which you move with the breath, can bring about energy and get you out of a funk.

However, if you are feeling heavy with exhaustion, the thought of doing any kind of movement might make you want to forsake the entire idea of yoga. At these times, it's important to meet yourself where you are and do resting poses, also known as restorative poses. Restorative poses are passive, easeful poses in which we support our bodies with props. They are designed to turn on the "relaxation response," also known as "rest and digest." If you find yourself drooling in a restful pose, you know you are doing it right.

Allowing yourself to just rest, in life or in yoga, can be scary. Some people feel if they "give in" to their exhaustion, they are giving up or letting themselves off the hook. They call themselves unproductive, selfish, or lazy. They say, in an apologetic tone, "I did a few restorative poses but no real yoga." But restorative yoga *is* real yoga—honoring the truth of what you need, resisting our society's pull to always be doing something, finding stillness. So invite yourself to enter a restorative pose with an attitude of friendliness and acceptance, getting yourself settled in as though you were tucking your child into bed.

I've noticed that when I begin a restorative pose, I always feel skeptical. I think, *I'm so tired—there's no way that in fifteen minutes I'll want to stand up again. I'll still feel groggy like I do after naps.* But almost every time, when fifteen minutes is up, I find myself renewed—my energy lighter and clearer.

Practice **Restorative Poses**

Here are two restorative poses that I love when I am exhausted:

Restorative Child's Pose
-   Have two yoga bolsters, OR a big couch cushion, OR a couple of pillows piled up.
-   Sit down with toes together, knees apart.
-   Bring one bolster or pillow out in front of you, in its longest orientation. Draw it in toward your belly. If pregnant, just bring it in to

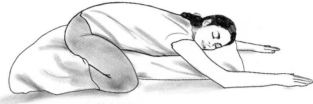

Child's Pose with props

your chest, leaving a little space for your belly. You can add extra pillows if you need more height. If you feel discomfort in your knees, sit on the other bolster or a few pillows.

-   Lie your torso down on the bolster or pillow in front of you, with your head facing one side. Arms can rest comfortably out to the sides. Stay here as long as you like, optimally for fifteen minutes. Halfway through, switch your head to face the other side.

-   If you have no props, you can still do child's pose. You just may not be able to stay as long comfortably. To do child's pose without props, sit with toes together, knees apart, and bring your head or chest down to the floor. Arms can stretch out in front of you or rest at your sides.

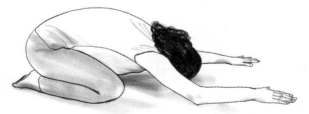

Child's Pose

Legs up the Wall

-   Bring your seat to the wall, lying down on your back, legs resting on the wall. Arms can be out to the side, on your belly, or (my favorite) up overhead holding opposite elbows. You may want to bring a bolster or pillow under your sacrum, especially if you are pregnant. Make sure that you position it so that it feels as comfortable as possible for your spine. You can support your head and neck with a folded blanket or small pillow.

- Another variation of this pose that I use almost every day with clients is "legs on the couch." It's just like legs up the wall, but in front of the couch. Let your lower legs be supported by the couch.

- Stay here as long as you like, optimally for fifteen minutes. If you are pregnant, lying on your back for too long may make you feel uncomfortable or out of breath, so a shorter amount of time might feel better.

Note: Though these poses can feel very luxurious, for someone who feels anxious they can be very tough. Stillness and rest can activate the worried mind. If you feel anxious and exhausted, consider preparing by doing some active poses or movement, like sun salutations, to get your anxious energy out before sinking into restorative yoga.

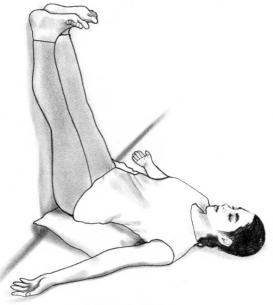

Legs Up on the Wall

I can't relax

Sometimes, you try to relax, and your nervous system won't calm down. Maybe your anxiety has been very high today. Maybe your baby has been crying for hours and your nerves are on edge. If you have PTSD, you may be in a state of hypervigilance, and it may be hard to let your guard down.

In Patanjali's *Yoga Sutras*, 1.34[16], he suggests a form of breathwork, *pranayama*, that is the key to finding calm: focus on lengthening the exhale. This yoga practice makes sense from a biological standpoint, too. Lengthening the exhale activates the parasympathetic nervous system, decreasing physiological arousal, slowing the heart rate, reducing blood pressure, and relaxing tightness in the body.

Many forms of *pranayama* invite us to lengthen the breath. Here are four that my clients seem to find most accessible:

Practice **Easy Rhythmic Breathing** (*Sukha Pranayama*)

Breathe to a count of 4. Count 4 for the inhale, and 4 for the exhale. If this feels doable, consider experimenting with 4 for the inhale and 6 for the exhale. If that works, you can see how it feels to try 4 for the inhale and 8 for the exhale.

Practice **OM**

An easier way to extend the exhale without having to count is to use your voice. When you make a sound with your voice, your breath comes out a bit more slowly than it does if you simply exhale.

At the beginning of many public yoga classes, the teacher will lead the class in chanting the sound of OM. There is a spiritual purpose for this sound, and the resonance of the voices in the room can create a peaceful feeling. But a big part of why that OM feels so good is that it causes a good, long exhale that calms you down and resets your nervous system, helping you transition from your busy day to your yoga practice.

Take a deep inhale, then chant a long OM: Aaaa-uuuu-mmmm, letting the sound come from your lower register. OM doesn't require you to remember any words, and can be both a release of energy and a soothing sound. When you are pregnant, your baby can feel the vibration of your voice in your body. Many moms have told me that chanting OM helped them through labor contractions, and helped calm their new babies when they were crying. When I teach Mom & Baby yoga, when the moms chant OM, all the babies often stop crying all at once—it's like magic!

Practice Bee Breath (Brahmari)

Bee breath is like chanting OM, but with your mouth closed.

Take a deep inhale, and then, with your mouth closed, make a sound on the exhale until you run out of breath. It's basically humming, and sounds like a buzzing bee. You can usually feel a strong vibration in your mouth. Some might find that to be a weird, uncomfortable feeling. Others might find it relaxing and focusing.

Traditionally, there is a specific mudra, or hand gesture, that goes with bee breath: *shanmukhi mudra.* If you'd like to try it, bring your hands to your face. Thumbs plug both ears. The other fingers rest over the eyes, with the tips of the middle fingers meeting at the center of the forehead. This mudra is also an excellent way to practice *pratyahara* or turning the senses inward. Many moms find it a relief, a way to shut the world out and go into a cozy cocoon, feeling deliciously alone. Others may find it induces a sense of being trapped or stuck. If it does that—skip it! You can also do half the mudra—just stick your thumbs in your ears, letting the other fingers rest on the forehead.

When you hum with your thumbs in your ears, you may notice that the vibration becomes much more intense, and for some, thus, much more relaxing.

Babies often find your bee breath soothing or, if they are older, hilarious! Toddlers may want to join in.

Practice Alternate Nostril Breathing

In *nadi shodana,* alternate nostril breathing, we inhale and exhale through one nostril and then the other. This sounds confusing and feels weird to most people at first. But it is the one breath practice that my clients find most consistently helpful. It's hard to worry or think of much else when you do this because it takes focus!

You may want to blow your nose before you start. If your nose is too stuffed for this to work, try leaving the mouth just a little bit open, so that it can share the work of the inhale with the nose.

Bring the right hand close to the face. Bring the pointer and middle fingers down to the palm. Slide the nose into the space between the ring finger and thumb. Press the thumb gently into the nose to close the right nostril. Exhale, then inhale through the left nostril. As you remove the thumb from the right nostril, use the ring finger to press gently into the nose, closing the left nostril. Exhale, then inhale through the right nostril. I often recommend repeating ten times, switching nostrils after each inhale.

No rest for the weary

I didn't call this book *Awake at 3 a.m.* for nothing. From pregnancy on into early parenthood, sleep is everything. Sleep deprivation can lead to anxiety and depression, and, reciprocally, these moods can make it hard to fall asleep or stay asleep. Because of these realities, when I work with a new mom, sleep is usually the very first issue we address. We ask 1) How is your baby sleeping? And 2) If your baby sleeps, what is your sleep like?

How is your baby sleeping?

For the first few months, you cannot, sadly, teach a baby to sleep. They eat often and regularly, and have not yet developed a biological rhythm of sleep and wake. Getting more sleep during this time, then, involves help from others. Consider asking your partner, a family member, or a postpartum doula to stay up with the baby in the middle of the night. Even an hour more of consecutive sleep can make a big difference in your mood, allowing you to be so much more present and connected with your baby than if you were exhausted.

If nighttime help is not possible, ask for help so you can take a day-time nap. I know they say "sleep when the baby sleeps," but without help, you may end up needing to use that time to eat, shower, or attend to an older child.

After a few months, you can consider setting up a sleep schedule for your baby. It can be a minefield reading about sleep online or in books. People have very strong opinions, both positive and nega-tive, about sleep training, cry-it-out, co-sleeping, and everything in between.

I remember reading that I should put my baby to bed "drowsy" but not asleep. This sounded great until I tried it, and my peaceful, drowsy baby would howl as soon as I put her down. I could only put her into bed after I nursed her until she passed out. I felt so guilty about not teaching her to fall asleep "properly," and I worried about her developing lifelong insomnia. It makes me sad to think that I felt stressed about that. Because a) I loved nursing her to sleep, and b) whoever came up with that idea had a child with a temperament that was very different from my baby's! In those early days, you have to do what works—and that means truly listening to your child and yourself.

For most moms I have worked with, some form of sleep training is essential to turning around PMADs. It can be hard to make it through the rough nights of sleep training, but in the end, parents and babies feel better rested, and moms report that their bond has actually improved.

For other moms I see, however, co-sleeping and breastfeeding on demand works better. Co-sleeping allows them to feed their babies without having to get up, walk into another room, and then rock a baby back to sleep. What do you think will work best for you? If it's hard to decide, sleep consultants, therapists, or pediatricians may be able to offer support or guidance.

If your baby sleeps, what is your sleep like? Can you let yourself rest? Can you fall and stay asleep?
Yoga therapy offers many tools for sleep:

- Turn on the relaxation response by making your sleeping space warm and dark, using extra pillows for comfort, and covering yourself with a nice, heavy blanket. If possible, keep electronic devices in another room, so that you associate your bed with sleep, not anxious Internet searches.
- Use mindful awareness to notice automatic thoughts like, *I can't function without sleep.* Getting rest is second best to getting sleep, so you can focus on rest instead of sleep.
- Forward folds can calm the nervous system, turn attention

inward, and promote sleep (page 187). You can practice forward folds before bed or whenever insomnia hits. I like to recommend poses you can do in bed! Child's pose and seated forward fold work well, and you can use pillows to support your head.

- Any breath practice in this book could help. Try a few and see what works for you.

- Body scan meditation, part of the yogic sleep practice, also known as yoga nidra, promotes rest and renewal.

Practice Body Scan

Body scan follows a very simple format. Many people practice by listening to a recording, which are available online (you can find one on my website). Listening enables you to totally let go of trying. Others like to guide themselves, doing the body scan at their own pace. Here are some basic instructions that you can lead yourself through silently.

In a body scan, you move your awareness through your body from head to toes. When each body part is named, you do not need to relax or change it in any way. Just let awareness dust over the area, lingering for a full breath, or as long as it feels interesting. If you fall asleep halfway through, wonderful.

Bring awareness to:
- Top of the head
- Scalp
- Ears
- Eyes and eyebrows—left, then right
- Nose, each nostril
- Mouth, inside and out
- Whole head
- Neck and throat
- Left arm—shoulder, upper arm, elbow, lower arm, hand, fingers

- Right arm—shoulder, upper arm, elbow, lower arm, hand, fingers
- Both arms at the same time
- Chest and upper back
- Belly
- Lower back
- Pelvis
- Seat
- Left leg—hip, thigh, knee, lower leg, foot, toes
- Right leg—hip, thigh, knee, lower leg, foot, toes
- Both legs at the same time
- Entire left side of the body
- Entire right side of the body
- Top of the body
- Bottom of the body
- Whole body

A moment alone

From the moment you are pregnant, you are not alone. You don't have the option to just do what you want to do, and feel the way you want to feel. Your every moment is affected by your baby. Many pregnant women feel as if their baby is a parasite—there every second, living off of your body!

After your baby is born, that doesn't change. Caring for a baby is a constant task. You rarely get a chance to go to the bathroom alone, to eat a meal in peace, or to get an idle hour to sit and be unproductive by yourself. Your baby is physically on your body for a lot of the day, too.

Early on, you may be desperate not to be alone. If you are alone with the baby all day, you might long for adult company. But over time, a fantasy of having some time just for yourself—without your baby—may emerge. This fantasy is worth listening to. Solitude can be the source of our deepest renewal, creativity, and spirituality.

It's very hard for most moms to seek out time alone. They might struggle to figure out the logistics, or feel guilty even wishing for it. Guilt can be especially potent for moms who are at work for most of the day. I hear moms say, "I'm away all day, I can't take any more time away from the baby."

Yet sometimes taking time alone is not only good for you, it is the best thing you can do for your baby, too. Wanting to be alone doesn't mean you don't love your baby or that you don't want to spend time with them. It just means you also want time alone.

When could you find time to be alone? Who could help make this happen? Your partner? A babysitter? What obstacles might come up? Are there financial concerns? Are you worried that someone will judge you or say no? Are you worried that someone else won't be as good at caring for your baby as you are?

Some great ways to be alone are:

- Go out somewhere in nature.
- Go for a walk.
- Send your family out to the grocery store.
- Sit in your car for a few minutes at the end of your work day before you go home.

You may also want time alone with your partner, maybe a night out together. Relationships need tending to, just as babies do. If you find yourself fighting with your partner or just growing distant, having some time alone together, without your baby, may be what you need to reconnect.

It can be helpful to think of the first few years of your child's life as an extension of pregnancy. You and the baby are one organism. You share nourishment and energy. Thus, just as in pregnancy, your caring for yourself *is* directly caring for your baby.

In yoga therapy, we often talk about each of us as having many layers of being, or *koshas*. We have the *annamaya kosha*, the physical layer; the *pranamaya kosha*, the energy layer; the *manomaya kosha*, the layer of thoughts and feelings; the *vijnanamaya kosha*, the layer of insight and wisdom; and the *anandamaya kosha*, the layer of bliss. You might think of how you and your baby are connected as relating to these sheaths.

In pregnancy, you and your baby are encircled by the same body, connected as one. At birth, and in the process of weaning, the baby slowly develops their own *annamaya kosha*, physical body. As they differentiate from you over the first few years, they slowly develop their own energy, their own thoughts and feelings, their own insight. I've heard it said that the last layer, the bliss body, separates into two on the child's third birthday, and then you become two separate people, capable of fully loving one another. I love this image. I picture a mother and baby in a golden sheath of light, thick at first and then thinner and more able to stretch and flow as time goes on, popping on the third birthday, raining down golden light on them both.

You and your baby are connected, so your connection remains, even when you take some time alone. Yes, leaving your baby might make them cry for a bit. When babies are little, separation is scary for them—they don't yet know you are not gone forever. But babies slowly develop *object permanence*, the understanding that an object still exists even if they can't see it. This is why they love to play peeka-boo—they find it thrilling to realize that you were there all along, even when a blanket was hiding your face.

Moms go through a parallel process of developing object perma-nence. Though we know our babies are physically still there when we don't see them, we worry that our connection with them falters, or that they won't know we love them unless we are right there. We slowly learn that these things are actually constant and unchanging.

When you trust that your connection remains intact, you allow the last sheath to dissolve, letting that golden light stay with each of you, right in your hearts.

Practice **Sound Meditation**

If you can't actually find time alone, you can practice *pratyahara*, turning inward. Sound meditation is a powerful way to turn inward in even the most intrusive of atmospheres.

Bring awareness to your ears, to sound coming into your ears. What can you hear that is the farthest away from you, in the wide world around you? Can you hear cars outside? Voices talking? Birds chirping?

Now bring awareness to sounds close by, perhaps in the room you are in. Can you hear machines buzzing? Sounds of other people close by? The building shifting?

Now bring awareness to sounds in your own body, perhaps your breath or your swallow. Maybe, if it is quiet enough, you can hear the sound of your own breathing. Now bring awareness to your inner self, deep within. Invite yourself to listen to what is in your mind and your heart. You may hear silence, or you may hear a symphony. Just notice, what do you hear when you listen carefully to yourself?

As you are ready to end this practice, invite back in each layer of sound, one by one, seeing if maybe just for a moment you can welcome in all the sounds at once.

Food struggles

Food is nourishment—emotionally and physically. It is the most basic form of caring for yourself and your baby. In yoga therapy, we think of eating as a relationship with food, asking not only *what* you eat, but also *how* you eat.

Thinking about "how" you eat encourages responsiveness—listening to your own body's needs. I once heard someone say, "No diet book, no lecture, no article, and not even your doctor can tell you whether or not you are hungry. Only your body can do that!" Yet there are so many things that get in the way of listening to our bodies, especially in pregnancy and new motherhood:

Body signals are off Your preferences, cravings, and aversions may be different. Sleep deprivation can mess with hunger and fullness signals. So can being too busy. If you skip eating all day while caring for your baby, your body may try to make up for it later by giving you urges to overeat.

Time When you are caring for a small baby, it is hard to have time to do anything, and it's easy for moms to put eating last on the list. Practically, someone has to buy groceries, prepare food, and clean the dishes—all of which can seem overwhelming. Eating while holding a baby can also make it hard to be present with your food and feel satisfied.

Rules Perhaps you've been told certain types of foods are "good" or "bad," or even "unsafe" for your baby or you. Perhaps you've been told that certain foods affect your milk and make your baby distressed. Or perhaps you have gestational diabetes and have to follow a restricted diet. Having specific food rules can be challenging and put food at the center of your attention. Especially if you have anxiety, food rules can become an obsession.

Stress Food can become a way of coping. You may overeat comfort foods or graze all day on treats, ignoring your nutrition needs.

Body image struggles Messages about the importance of losing "baby weight" or comments from others about your body can lead you to ignore body signals.

With all of these challenges, you may need to use deliberate tools to help you listen to your body. Here are some attitudes and behaviors to help encourage responsiveness to your body's needs:

Let go of judging foods There is no one right diet. Try to let go of the idea of "good" foods and "bad" foods. Nutrition science is always changing, so let your body be your guide, instead of what you read in an article. Think about what would make your own body feel good *and* what would taste good.

Have food available It can be hard to stop eating when you are full. This is because listening to hunger cues often needs to come first. Ignoring hunger signals because you don't think you "should" eat makes all of your body's signals more confusing. Eat when you are hungry. If you let your body know you will eat when it sends hunger signals, your fullness signals will be easier and easier to follow.

Eat "good enough" food It's okay to ask friends to bring meals or help prep food, and to eat foods that are frozen, microwaved, prepared, or just not as perfect as you would like. Better to eat something good enough when you are hungry than to wait for something perfect. Make a list of quick foods that you can have on hand—and that you can eat with one hand! Include foods with different colors, textures, and tastes to help you feel satisfied. Try to eat at least every four hours when you are awake.

Practice body acceptance Your body made a baby, and this causes bodies to change. Breastfeeding also affects your body. Some people lose pregnancy weight right away; some never do. People who lose weight immediately aren't fake, and people who don't lose weight aren't lazy. They just have different bodies—all bodies are different.

Let go of weight loss as a goal Working to lose weight now (or any time, for that matter) is a drain on energy and on self-worth.

If you need some more help or advice, consider seeing a registered dietitian or therapist who specializes in Intuitive Eating for moms. If you have a history of disordered eating, be extra gentle, careful, and aware of your relationship with food, and check in with your support team. Hormonal changes, body changes, stress, and food prep challenges can trigger relapse. This is a very vulnerable time.

Practice **Mindful Eating**

Mindful eating means paying attention to the act of eating—noticing thoughts, feelings, and sensations, and eating in a way that feels intentional, instead of rushed and unsatisfying. Try taking at least one mindful bite of food at the beginning of each meal.

Pause before you begin. Notice how you feel in your body. Look at your food and notice the colors and textures. Smell your food. As you lift the food up to take your first bite, notice how your mouth reacts—if it begins to water, how it opens. Put food in your mouth, then put your fork down. Sometimes we have an urge to start putting more food on our fork before we have finished the bite we are on. Notice that urge and return the attention back to the bite in your mouth. Notice how the food feels on your tongue. Notice how the taste buds react. Notice how the tongue moves the food around your teeth while you chew. Notice what you smell as you eat. Continue to chew your food with awareness. When you swallow, pay attention to what urges come up next, and pause just one more moment to notice before you take your next bite.

Breastfeeding

Breastfeeding can have many wonderful benefits for mom and baby, providing nutrition, boosting immunity, helping with bonding, and releasing oxytocin, a feel-good hormone.

Breastfeeding can, however, be a source of shame, self-criticism, obsession, and grief for many moms, and that's important to acknowledge. It can be fraught with pain and endless worries about milk supply, engorgement, or whether something you ate is giving your baby gas. It can be hard to find spaces that feel comfortable or welcoming to nurse or pump outside of your home. If this is your experience, please offer yourself compassion and words of encouragement. You are doing a brave, beautiful, and difficult thing for yourself and your baby!

Moms may hear another mom say, "I almost stopped breastfeeding, it was so hard, but I kept trying and then it got easier!" You may hear this and think you aren't trying hard enough. Moms sometimes feel that they have failed as a parent, as a woman, or as a human if they don't breastfeed. They may stay up day and night pumping endlessly, desperate for each ounce. They may hide while feeding their babies with a bottle in public, or apologize for using formula.

I've also heard moms with PMADs say they feel that breastfeeding is the only good thing they can do for their baby. But what babies truly need is your love. Breastfeeding is just one of many meaningful ways of bonding and being of service to your baby. You are more than a milk provider!

For many moms with PMADs, getting regular sleep is one of the most important parts of recovery. This may mean that you decide to let your partner or another caregiver feed your baby at night so you can sleep.

If this brings up self-criticism, remind yourself:

- My baby is getting really good nourishment.
- I am taking care of myself, which is an essential part of taking care of my baby.
- Breastfeeding is great, and bottle-feeding is great, too.
- My baby gets to bond with their other parent.

I don't suggest saying to yourself, "Well, I worked hard, but this is the best I could do," or "I can at least feel good that I tried." This implies that by bottle-feeding, you are doing something wrong, which you are not. You, too, are doing a brave, beautiful, and difficult thing for yourself and your baby!

Some moms feel both a deep love and joy in breastfeeding, and also significant stress trying to make it work. If you experience this kind of stress, consider getting support: a lactation consultant (LC) can be a true lifesaver. LCs can help you come up with practical, individualized plans for dealing with latch, pain, milk supply, and more. LCs can also help you stop judging yourself, feel less alone, feel more hope, and reduce anxiety.

When you are in a tender place, however, sometimes something an LC says may feel triggering. Breastfeeding can be such a sensitive topic, and the job of LCs means they jump between the oft-conflicting roles of teacher, cheerleader, and empathic counselor. The skills can feel impractical or overwhelming, or the cheerleading overbearing. Moms often worry about letting down the LC if they don't "succeed" at breastfeeding. Remember that they are just humans (usually very kind ones!), and they are most helpful when you speak up for yourself and take just the tips that work for you.

Whether you bottle-feed or breastfeed, feeding your baby can be a wonderful opportunity to meditate. In the first few weeks, feeding might be complicated or painful as you get the hang of it. But as you settle into your rhythm of feeding, meditation can become more possible. No pressure, of course—feeding can also be a time to read, talk to others, watch TV, coo at your baby, or close your eyes and zone out. But, if you are looking for an easy time to sit yourself down and meditate, this is a good one.

Practice Feeding Meditation

As you sit with your baby, focus on the sensations of the feeding or nursing experience. You will find some of these sensations pleasant and some unpleasant. See if you can note these without judging yourself as good or bad for your reactions. When your mind wanders, gently bring yourself back to the sensations:

- The weight of your baby on your arms or lap
- The warmth of your baby
- The softness of your baby's skin or hair
- The pattern of their breath
- The sounds your baby makes as they eat
- If nursing, the sensation of baby suckling on your nipple and of your breasts making milk and then emptying
- If bottle-feeding, the sensation and sound of baby suckling on the bottle, how the suckling pulls the bottle a bit in your hand
- If your baby is awake, awareness of seeing their eyes and feeling their movements as they stroke, kick, and poke you

Exercise

Exercise has been shown to help with PMADs, and mood in general.[17] Regular cardiovascular exercise can sometimes even be as effective as antidepressants in changing brain chemistry. Unfortunately, since some key features of depression are a lack of motivation and a feeling of inertia, finding the wherewithal to exercise can be as challenging as healing depression itself!

It's even harder to exercise when you are pregnant and feel nauseated, uncomfortable, in pain, or unwieldy. It's also hard to exercise with a new baby. Your body probably feels totally different—and you've lost physical strength and endurance. Maybe you have some ongoing pain or injury after childbirth, or your pelvic floor is weak and you leak urine when you walk. Yup—all these things are totally legitimate reasons to not feel like moving.

The good news is that exercise to help with your mood does not have to be dramatic. A walk counts. And—yoga asana counts! Anything that gets your blood flowing, increases your heart rate, and encourages your body to send out hormones that make you feel good (endorphins) works.

From a yogic point of view, movement shifts your energy. If your PMAD has a heavy, depressed quality, movement is thought to "break up" that heaviness, to bring in lightness and spaciousness. If you are feeling anxious, movement is thought to release or use up some of your anxious energy, leaving room for you to feel calm. Either way, you cultivate internal and external strength, a sense of competence, and endurance for the marathon that is parenting a baby.

You might think you need to really push yourself to follow a challenging exercise routine. But, paradoxically, pushing yourself too hard can actually make it difficult to keep up with an exercise routine. If you decide that exercise has to look like it did before you were pregnant, or that it has to be running or weight lifting or require a certain kind of clothing, you may be able to force yourself a few times, but over time, you will start to resist it. You may also injure yourself, which for sure makes it hard to exercise!

You might also think that it will help motivate you to focus on a goal of weight loss. However, this, too, actually gets in the way of regular movement. When people exercise for weight loss, they tend to stop doing it over time. Perhaps this is because they become demoralized when they don't lose the amount of weight they'd hoped to. People are more likely to stick to an exercise routine when their primary motivation is to improve their mood and well-being.[18]

Here are some things you can do to help make it easier on yourself:

- Keep a yoga mat out on the floor or easily accessible.
- Keep sneakers or slip-on walking shoes by your door.
- Make a plan with a friend or family member to go for a walk.
- Set small, realistic goals—you do not need to set a goal to take five yoga classes a week. Or even one yoga class a week. Maybe your goal is just to do five sun salutations a day.
- Set a schedule . . . and be willing to change it. Having a routine makes it easier to fight past inertia. Once a baby comes, however, you might have a plan to go for a walk, and your baby poops all over you. If this happens, say to yourself with compassion, "It's okay that I'm not going to go for a walk right now. Stuff happens. As soon as I change this diaper I'll make a plan for when I can do it later." Maybe it won't be till after the next nap, or maybe not until tomorrow. But resist the urge to either berate yourself or give up.

Most important, choose a form of movement that you like (or at least that you don't hate)! Find a way to move that brings you pleasure by getting you outside, making you listen to music, or connecting you with others.

Practice **Sun Salutations**

There are countless ways to do sun salutations. You might already know a favorite flow that you've practiced for years. Maybe that works now, or maybe you have to accommodate it for the body you have today. I'll share a version here that can be practiced in pregnancy and as soon as you feel ready postpartum. First, we will go over downward-facing dog pose and plank pose.

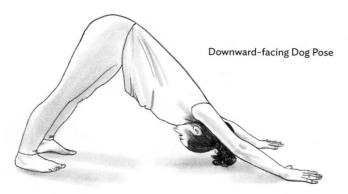

Downward-facing Dog Pose

Downward-facing Dog Pose
- Start in standing forward fold (page 187)
- Bend the knees a lot, bringing the hands to the floor, shoulder-distance apart, with the middle fingers pointing forward.
- Press the fingers, knuckles, and palms into the ground firmly, spreading the fingers wide.
- Keeping hips high, step the feet back about 3 to 4 feet behind you, so that you are in an upside-down V. Work toward a straight line from your hands up to your tailbone. Feet stay roughly hip-distance apart, and heels move in the direction of the ground. They do not need to reach the ground. Head and neck are soft and released.

- If you have any rounding or discomfort in your back, you can bend the knees a lot. The legs do not need to be straight.
- Focus the energy on pressing through the hands, finding openness through the armpits, and increasing the spaciousness and stability in your back.

Plank Pose

- From downward-facing dog, keep the hands planted, and bring the shoulders forward so that they are right over the wrists. Hips come down a bit so that you are no longer in a V, but instead, the whole torso and legs are like a plank of wood, one straight line from head to heels. You may need to step the feet slightly back to do this. The abdominal muscles hug gently in to support you.

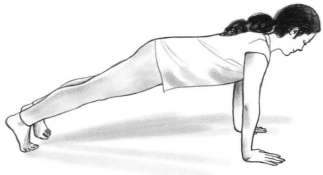

Plank

- During pregnancy and the postpartum period, it can be a good idea to go a little bit easier on the abdominal muscles by doing a version of plank we will call "plank on knees" (see following page). In this version, as you bring shoulders forward from downward-facing dog, bring the knees to the ground. Drop the hips slightly, so that the long straight line of the plank is now from the head to the knees.

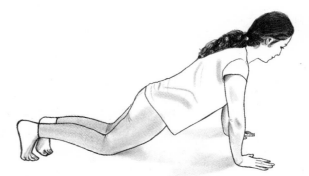

Plank on Knees

Sun salutation for pregnancy and postpartum
Sun salutations can be done quickly, with just one or two breaths for each pose. For exercise, I like to do at least five in a row. Move with the breath, inhaling as you enter each pose, exhaling as you exit it.

- Mountain pose (page 91)
- Mountain pose with arms reaching up
- Standing forward fold (pagse 187)
- Downward-facing dog
- Plank on knees
- Plank on knees with elbows bent back a few inches (as if you are lowering yourself toward the floor)
- Plank on knees with backbend: straighten arms, broaden collarbones into upper body backbend, hips stay in plank alignment
- Downward-facing dog
- Standing forward fold
- Mountain pose

If you forget a movement or add one in, it's fine! Just play with linking up the breath and the movement and enjoying the flow.

I can't handle this

PMADs are often marked by intense self-doubt. It can be hard to trust yourself in any way when you think poorly of yourself. In my own dark moments, I noticed I would often say, "I can't handle this." I said it to my husband, repeatedly. I said it to my friends. I said it to myself. Saying it served a purpose—it was a way of communicating how terrible I felt and, in a roundabout way, asking to be saved.

But it had two negative consequences: it eroded my sense of trust in myself, and it sometimes eroded the trust my husband had in me. When he couldn't save me, I felt angry. And when he let me off the hook and took over something that I had told him that I couldn't handle, I felt hurt that he didn't trust my strength. (Poor guy—couldn't win!)

Many of us struggle our whole lives with trusting ourselves and our bodies. Then, if you had a hard time getting pregnant or suffered a loss, you may have lost any trust in your body that you did have. If you felt sick in pregnancy, you might have felt betrayed—why would your body do this to you? If your baby has colic, and you expected to have the "maternal instincts" to meet their needs, you might have lost trust in your ability to be a mom. If you develop PMADs, your trust in yourself and your strength might really be shaken.

Birth is another occasion when trust becomes challenged. First, in medical settings, sometimes the mom's body is the last thing professionals trust. Birth can be forced to happen on a schedule, or in a certain way, or a certain position. Often (though not always), a woman is not "allowed" to start pushing, even when her body has the urge, unless the provider tells her that she is dilated enough.

But, conversely, I worry a lot about how many holistic perinatal professionals, and especially we prenatal yoga teachers, talk about "trusting your body" during pregnancy and birth. I wish, instead, we used language like "*listen to your body*" or, my favorite, "*respond to your body.*"

If a woman says she trusts her body, and everything turns out the way she wanted it, what a wonderful blessing! But in my time as a prenatal yoga teacher and psychotherapist (and as a friend), I have known hundreds of women who deeply trusted their bodies in birth, who had a strong, grounded awareness of their body and soul's wholeness and fullness, who had calm, open, presence—and who still experienced their birth or their early days with a new baby as very different from what they had hoped or intended.

Many of these moms feel traumatized by the fact that their trust didn't pan out, perhaps feeling betrayed by their bodies, or as though they had failed. They might feel especially alienated, in a subsequent pregnancy, by a prenatal yoga teacher or a well-meaning friend telling them to trust their bodies.

In pregnancy and afterward, it is essential to find a deeper form of trust than just trusting we will get a happy outcome. Trusting yourself doesn't have to mean that everything will go your way; it means trusting that you have an unchanging inner steadiness that can greet whatever comes your way.

Over time, I have learned that when I feel overwhelmed, I can honor both my difficult feeling and my trust in myself by saying, "This feels overwhelming. It's hard. I can ask for help figuring out how to get through it." I marshal the support that I need and invite my partner to be just that—my partner, my teammate—instead of my savior. I learn to trust my coping skills, my ever-present breath, my use of my voice, my perseverance, and our collective problem-solving abilities.

It's also important to note that trusting yourself doesn't mean that you must reject trusting others. It may mean that you trust your ability to pick wise advisors, to hear them out, and to sift through and experiment with their advice.

In my training to be a therapist, one of the first things I remember learning is that you should never say to a client, "You can trust me," or "This is a safe space for you." We as therapists have to *earn* the trust of our clients and establish a sense of safety with our actions. The same goes for you—you have to earn your own trust. This can be hard when you haven't shown up for yourself in the past—when you've checked out with compulsive behaviors, avoided things that are meaningful to you, or told yourself how worthless, weak, or terrible you are.

We can rebuild trust by acting in a trustworthy way toward ourselves. Perhaps this means showing up to take care of ourselves by eating, sleeping, and resting as much as we need to. Perhaps this means talking to ourselves in a kind and encouraging manner. Perhaps this means asking for help or facing our fears.

Developing mastery over new tasks can also help. I have a master's degree and a successful career, but in my postpartum sleep-deprived and hormonal state, I felt completely bewildered and overwhelmed when I had to figure out how to operate a breast pump. What tasks seem bewildering or overwhelming to you? Perhaps it's how to find childcare or put together a work schedule, how to swaddle, or how to set up your baby's health insurance.

Choose one task to take on. Consider asking someone who has mastered this task before to help you—one of my sweetest memories of being a new mama was having a friend with a baby a few weeks older come and teach me and my husband how to use our baby wrap carrier. Take it one step at a time. Practice. Notice how it feels over time. How does it affect your depression or anxiety to gain a sense of mastery, even over something small?

Building a steady yoga practice, in which we show up with gentle awareness for ourselves and do the poses, meditation, or breathwork we committed to, even when we feel like a total mess, is another way to build trust. You learn that you can trust yourself to show up no matter what.

Practice **Mastery**

Pick a somewhat challenging pose that you'd like to explore. Keep-ups
(page 117), standing forward fold (page 187), warrior II (page 79), or tree pose
(page 92) could all work. Greet the pose every day in your practice. Notice,
over time, how your ability to stay in the pose grows. Perhaps you find that
you started out holding the pose for three breaths, but over time, you are
able to hold the pose for ten breaths. Perhaps you notice that you develop
greater stability in the pose, or greater openness. Perhaps you feel more and
more able to release tension in tight muscles. Perhaps you develop your
sense of alignment in the pose. Bring mindfulness to the changes, developing
awareness of your ability to slowly grow and change, even in the face of a
challenge. And the great thing about yoga is that—while you never truly
master a pose—as you become more comfortable, you can grow into new
variations!

Trauma

Trauma is defined as experiencing, witnessing, or being exposed to something that threatens life, safety, or well-being. You can experience trauma with something that happens to you or with something that happens to your loved ones.

If a mom has experienced trauma in childbirth, or from past loss, or from her own childhood, she may find that she feels scared often. She may have intrusive memories or nightmares. She may be "hyper-vigilant"—her nervous system constantly in a state of stress, her mind scanning her environment for danger. Or she might feel numb, as if it is hard to be present in her body. Others may not understand why she feels this way, especially if nothing bad is happening right now.

All these symptoms are actually her mind and body's way of protecting her, trying to prevent bad things from happening again. Her body learns from trauma and does its best to keep her safe. In psychology, we often say that post-traumatic stress is a "normal reaction to abnormal circumstances."

Key to healing from trauma and finding a feeling of safety is to give yourself new experiences, through which your body, not just your mind, can learn that it is safe. A good place to start is by focusing on *choice*. You do not have to accept every single thing that happens to you. You can practice saying no, asking for what you want, letting your needs be known.

In pregnancy, choice is especially important. For moms with a trauma history, having a birth plan is a good start. Even though you cannot plan for how the labor will go, you can let everyone around you know how you want to be treated. You can collaborate with your care providers to make sure that anyone at your birth knows, for example, how important it is to you that every intervention be carefully explained, that no one touch you without your permission, or that unnecessary vaginal exams be avoided.

Yoga classes are a good place to experiment with choice. In most yoga classes, the teacher dictates what the poses should look like, and students feel compelled to do what the teacher says. But you don't have to! I don't recommend that you go to a yoga class and just do your own thing. But if a teacher tells you to do something and it hurts or makes you feel anxious or triggered, you can choose to stop or modify in a way that feels good to you. Same thing goes for if a teacher touches you in yoga class to give you an assist or adjustment—you can tell them if you don't want to be touched right then, or ever.

It's important to find a yoga teacher who honors your choices. If you have trouble finding one, keep looking. You can always walk out of a class that doesn't feel right.

Years ago, I took a yoga workshop with a famous teacher, whose method was to focus on how the "issues are in the tissues," doing extensive "hip openers," which were supposed to "release" trauma. During one part of the class, it became too hot and intense for me, and I felt dizzy. I sat down and closed my eyes for a few moments, waiting until I felt more grounded. The teacher came over and, in front of a room of eighty people, chastised me for "shutting down" and urged me to "find my strength." I left the room shaking and holding back tears, with more trauma in my body than I came in with.

A week later, I was in class with a local teacher. His classes were also quite intense, took place in a heated room, and involved very challenging postures. Because of what had happened with the other teacher, I felt intimidated and hesitant. What would he do to me if I needed to rest again?

After we began moving, the student next to me entered child's pose. She stayed in child's pose for the whole class. I became perplexed and preoccupied, wondering what she was doing. I looked over again and again to see if the teacher would come over and berate her. At the end of class, the teacher stopped and asked us all to draw our attention to this student, for she, in honoring her body, had practiced true *ahimsa*, non-harming, and had demonstrated the most advanced practice in the room that day.

Take his message to heart. It is not a cop-out to listen to your body or to make a personal choice in a yoga class—or anywhere else, for that matter. It is a sign of an advanced practice, of willingness to let go of comparing and just be yourself.

Practice **Choice in Yoga with Neck Stretch**

- Sit in a comfortable position.
- Lean your head to the left, bringing the left ear in the direction of the shoulder.
- Notice what happens with the left shoulder. If it lifts, you may want to experiment with softening it back down and seeing if you like that.
- Next, bring awareness to the right side of the neck, noticing what the sensation of the stretch feels like. You can experiment with turning the chin down a bit to see how that changes the stretch. Then you may want to experiment with turning the chin up. Find the position of the head that you choose to stay with.
- Another choice you could make would be to lift the left hand up and over the scalp, so it rests on the right ear, gently pulling the head a bit more to the left. If you like how it feels, you can leave it there. You can also make a choice to let the hand fall back down if you don't like it.
- When you are done in the stretch, bring your left hand to the left cheek and use the strength of your hand to guide your head back to an upright position, perhaps noticing the difference in feeling on the two sides of the neck. When you are ready, you can take the other side.

When maternal instincts don't kick in

In our culture, we have a collective fairy tale in which, at the moment of birth, a magical spell comes over a mother, and something called the "maternal instinct" kicks in. In real life, however, many moms feel no such thing. They feel lost and confused, as if someone forgot to hand them the baby manual. They might feel ashamed to admit, "I don't know what I'm doing." But not knowing what you are doing is normal, and needn't be something to beat yourself up for. Parenting does not come "naturally" to many of us, especially if we didn't grow up in families where there were a lot of babies around.

You'll hear a lot of people say, "Don't listen to anyone, because you are the expert on your baby." That's silly. You are not the expert on your baby. It takes years to become an expert on anything. And your baby is changing and new every day. This is like visiting a new country and assuming you should already know exactly how to speak the language, follow customs, and navigate the subway.

You are not an expert on your baby, and no one else is either. But the good news is: you don't have to be! Being an expert gets in the way of responsiveness, flexibility, and accepting help from others. It leads to comparisons and shoulds. Instead of trying to be a "good mother" or an expert, what if we focused on being a mom who is ready to experiment, see her child as they are, and keep growing?

"Beginner's mind" is a mindful attitude we can cultivate with curiosity to help us parent as we are today, maternal instinct or no maternal instinct. It means pausing and saying, with no shame, "I don't know what I'm doing." It means taking the risk of trying on paradigm shifts, letting go of old ways of understanding and opening up to new ones. And then doing that again.

It's too bad in prenatal and postnatal yoga classes when moms focus on the way they used to be able to do poses, as though that was better or more advanced yoga. The judgment means they are missing what the poses have to teach them in this body, right now.

I have felt some of these things, too—I am occasionally sad that I will likely never do a bird-of-paradise pose again. But what I have found is that losing my old relationship with poses gave me the gift of finding beginner's mind without trying. Life is a good yoga teacher that way. I get to feel the joy of discovery in poses that I remember loving from my first year of practice—figuring out where to flex my toes, rotate my hip, or lengthen my spine to feel just a little bit more steadiness or spaciousness.

I show up at yoga class now, and instead of feeling that I am there to perform or test out my strength and flexibility, I am just there as a beginner—open to play, experiment, and delight in my body as it moves.

My children teach me beginner's mind, too! Whenever I've mastered the best "mindful parenting" technique to deal with their anxiety, or their temper tantrums, or their middle-of-the-night wake-ups, they humble me again. They teach me that I need to keep trying new things, that different things work for each of them, at different ages, on different days. They teach me that I don't always have to know what to do—often I just have to love them and they figure out what they need on their own.

One of my favorite beginner's mind moments was with my younger daughter, around age two, who was crying and crying. I kept trying to find ways to soothe her, letting her know that I was there, rocking her, offering to read a book, to give her a bath, to sing a song, to let her take a break. I offered all the things my instincts gave me, and everything I thought I knew about what soothed her. And then, when I gave up, stopped trying to be the expert, and just sat there open to learning, she transformed into my teacher, saying, "Mama! I just need to cry in your arms. For a long time."

Practice **Beginner's Eyes**

My family and I live steps away from a forest, so we are lucky to be able to hike often. When my younger daughter was an infant, I would put her into a carrier and hike there almost every day. She became deeply familiar with the smell, sights, and climate of the forest. One day, when she was eighteen months old, deep into a family hike, she said, "Out!" over and over until we decided to take her out of the carrier and let her start walking with us.

She walked quickly at first, keeping pace with the family, enjoying her newfound independence. Then she came across a small stick on the ground that crossed her path. She stopped and stooped down to look at it. She looked at it for about thirty seconds, then touched it, caressed it, picked it up, threw it, and squealed with joy. Then, to our amazement and amusement, she got all the way down on the ground and kissed it. She sat up and smiled. She looked around her. She saw another stick a few feet away and walked over, got down on the ground again, and kissed that one.

She went on like this for a few minutes, as though she were enacting some kind of primal earth worshiping ritual. My husband, older daughter, and I watched her enjoying the earth from a state of true beginner's mind. We all noticed and stood in awe of the beauty of the forest floor that we would have missed hiking at our usual pace.

Children can be our greatest guides into the realm of beginner's mind, encouraging us to see things through fresh eyes. We can call this way of literally seeing new details in the world around us "beginner's eyes." You can practice beginner's eyes anywhere—in the room you sit in now, at your doctor's office, on the bus, in nature, and sitting with your children.

Beginner's Eyes Right Now

Look at the room around you. Find an everyday object that you could practice seeing with "beginner's eyes." Imagine that you are an alien from Mars and you've never seen this object before. Touch it, move it, smell it, look at it in different lights. Explore and describe it without prior knowledge. For example, if you pick up a pen, you might describe it as "hard and non-porous, a tube with something inside, the length of my hand, has a point on the end that black stuff comes out of if you touch it."

Beginner's Eyes in Nature
Go outside. Find a leaf or a flower, and pretend that it is the first time you've seen it. Watch the sunset, reminding yourself that you don't know what colors will show up next, curious about what will happen.

Beginner's Eyes with Your Baby
Sit and look at your baby. Remind yourself that your baby is different today than they were yesterday. Look at their hands—they are only this exact size once! What do you notice? What's changing?

Conclusion

I chose to end the book with the practice of beginner's mind because this is the attitude I hope you walk away with at the end of this book. Do not expect yourself to have mastered yoga, erased your anxiety, conquered your depression, or become a perfect parent by the time you finish reading this, by the time your baby turns one, or even in this lifetime. I hope you put down this book feeling like you can begin again at any moment, that you won't judge how your practice "works" by how good you have become, but, instead, by how many times you are willing to awaken, open your mind, and reconnect to yourself and your family.

I hope that, in your darkest times, you have found a bit more of the quality known in yoga as *sattva*, the light of awakening.

Sattvic light does not mean happiness, bliss, or positivity. You might think of it as a flashlight illuminating something you couldn't see before. This light allows you to see your suffering with clarity and peace instead of judgment. Some signs that you are welcoming more light in are:

- You witness, acknowledge, and welcome your suffering, ask for help, and let others help you.
- You let go of being a perfect mom, and just let yourself, your baby, and your family do what you need to do to get through the day.
- You take steps to care for yourself even when you feel bad— working to get more rest, eat well, and love your baby in a way that feels grounded.
- You know that you will get through this.

I hope you walk away feeling a bit softer toward yourself, understanding that you are not bad, crazy, or selfish. I hope you feel comforted that you are not alone. I hope you have some new tools to care for your body, to build your strength, endurance, and flexibility to get through both your journey of mothering and your journey of healing. I hope you find compassion for your humanness and a willingness to meet the needs of your body, mind, and heart—for your well-being, for your family's well-being, and for the light you can bring to our greater community. I hope you have discovered a connection to your breath, your awareness, and your true, unchanging nature that you can come back to whenever times get tough. I hope that each day, you wake up again to what is really happening, to see and feel yourself and your baby as brilliant specks of light in this beautiful mess of existence.

I hope that you walk away with hope.

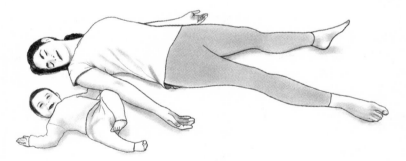

Savasana with baby

Notes

1   Katherine L. Wisner, et al. "Onset Timing, Thoughts of Self-Harm, and Diagnoses in Postpartum Women with Screen-Positive Depression Findings," *JAMA Psychiatry,* 2013; 70(5): 490–498. doi:10.1001/jama-psychiatry.2013.87
     http://www.who.int/mental_health/maternal-child/maternal_mental_health/en/

     https://www.marchofdimes.org/pregnancy/postpartum-depression.aspx

2   Wisner et al., "Onset"; Carla L. DeSisto , Shin Y. Kim, and Andrea J. Sharma. "Prevalence Estimates of Gestational Diabetes Mellitus in the United States, Pregnancy Risk Assessment Monitoring System (PRAMS), 2007–2010." *Preventing Chronic Disease* (2014): 11. https://www.cdc.gov/pcd/issues/2014/13_0415.htm

3   Leo Tolstoy, *Anna Karenina,* trans. Rosamund Bartlett (Oxford: Oxford University Press, 2016).

4   "Postpartum Depression Facts," National Institute of Mental Health, https://www.nimh.nih.gov/health/publications/postpartum-depression-facts/index.shtml

5   Wisner et al., "Onset."

6   Amy Weintraub, *Yoga for Depression: A Compassionate Guide to Relieving Suffering through Yoga* (New York: Broadway Books, 2004).

7   Swami Satchidananda, *The Yoga Sutras of Patanjali* (Yogaville, VA: Integral Yoga Publications, 2012).

8   Marsha M. Linehan, *DBT Skills Training Manual,* second edition (New York: Guilford Press, 2014).

9   Joanne V. Wood, W. Q. Elaine Perunovic, and John W. Lee, "Positive Self-Statements: Power for Some, Peril for Others," *Psychological Science* (0956-7976) 20, no. 7 (2009): 860–866. Psychology and Behavioral Sciences Collection, EBSCOhost (accessed September 23, 2017).

10   Satchidananda, *Yoga Sutras.*

11 Marjo Flykt, Katri Kanninen, Jari Sinkkonen, and Raija-Leena Punamäki, "Maternal Depression and Dyadic Interaction: The Role of Maternal Attachment Style," *Infant and Child Development* 19, no. 5 (2010): 530–550. Psychology and Behavioral Sciences Collection, EBSCOhost (accessed October 1, 2017); Barbara A. Bettes, "Maternal Depression and Motherese: Temporal and Intonational Features," *Child Development* 59, no. 4 (1988): 1089. SocINDEX with Full Text, EBSCOhost (accessed October 1, 2017).

12 Satchidananda, *Yoga Sutras*.

13 Fredrickson, Barbara L., Stephanie M. Noll, Tomi-Ann Roberts, Diane M. Quinn, and Jean M. Twenge. 1998. "That Swimsuit Becomes You: Sex Differences in Self-Objectification, Restrained Eating, and Math Performance." *Journal Of Personality & Social Psychology* 75, no. 1: 269-283. SocINDEX with Full Text, EBSCOhost (accessed December 17, 2017).

14 Lisa R. Rubin and Julia R. Steinberg, "Self-Objectification and Pregnancy: Are Body Functionality Dimensions Protective?" *Sex Roles* (2011): 65:606–618. DOI 10.1007/s11199-011-9955-y

15 Jennifer Daubenmier, "The Relationship of Yoga, Body Awareness, and Body Responsiveness to Self-Objectification and Disordered Eating," *Psychology of Women Quarterly*, 29 (2005), 207–219.

16 Satchidananda, *Yoga Sutras*.

17 Deborah Da Costa, et al. "A Randomized Clinical Trial of Exercise to Alleviate Postpartum Depressed Mood," *Journal of Psychosomatic Obstetrics and Gynecology*, September 2009; 30(3): 191–200.

18 David K. Ingledew and David Markland, "The Role of Motives in Exercise Participation," *Psychology and Health*, 23, no. 7 (2008).

Acknowledgments

Thank you to Jen Kamenetz, my original acquisitions editor, for inviting and encouraging me to write this book. At the time, I had no idea I could do such a thing, particularly with two small kids, and you gave me the gift of discovering how much I enjoy writing.

Thank you to Jess Beebe, my amazing and talented developmental editor, another person without whom this book would not exist. Your thoughtful and intelligent feedback brought clarity to what I hoped to say, amplified my messages, helped me uncover and feel good about my writing voice, and created the shape of this book. You and your Post-it notes saved me from giving up! What you did for me is what I aspire to do as a therapist: you helped me see where I needed to make changes without ever making me feel criticized; you made me feel deeply understood and empowered; and instead of just giving me answers, you guided me toward finding my own.

Thank you to the team at Parallax. To Hisae Matsuda, for your encouragement and open-mindedness as the focus of this book kept shape-shifting. Thank you for holding a light up to what I wanted one of the most salient messages of the book to be—that our job isn't to fix or create our children, it is just to love them. To Jacob Surpin, for stepping in as an editor late in the game and guiding me through each final stage with enthusiasm, kindness, ease, and wisdom. To Terri Saul, for your patience with my obsessive aesthetics and your hard work toward finding a perfect cover.

Thanks to Alexandra Bowman for a more beautiful cover than I could ever have imagined. I first saw Alexandra's artwork on the most inspiring poster, a vision of intersectional feminism, that I saw at the Women's March in Oakland. Having your art on this book is a bit of a dream come true. Thank you to Sara Christian for creating the lovely illustrations found in the book on an impossible deadline, all with an attitude of thoughtfulness and enthusiasm.

Thank you to Kylie Gordon (and little Lilou Krubiner) for posing for the illustrations, gracing this book and all the women who read it with your loving mama presence. I love you and our (almost twenty-year!) friendship so much, and my appreciation of your brilliance, compassion, realness, warmth, and beauty only deepens each year.

Thank you to Steve and Doreen Maller for lending me your sanctuary of a home, surrounded by nature, for my writer's retreat, as well as for your friendship for many years. Your home is an alchemical place where this book finally found its heart and soul.

In yoga, it is customary to honor one's teachers, and Jane Austin is at the top of my list. I practiced yoga for more than ten years before I got to study with her, and yet I think everything I know about yoga, I learned from her. Jane, thank you for your love and wisdom—for being a teacher and role model in both yoga and motherhood. I miss your classes so much that I sometimes contemplate getting pregnant again just so I can take them again! I recommend anyone reading this check out Jane's online classes, which you can find through her website at janeaustinyoga.com.

Thank you to BK Bose and the teachers at the Niroga Institute, for providing a solid foundation in yoga therapy. I especially want to thank Antonia Fokken, my yoga therapy mentor, for teaching me how to combine my two loves, yoga and therapy. Antonia, your wisdom, kindness, and faith in me are a big part of how I ended up writing this book.

I also want to honor the three yoga and mindfulness teachers with whom I studied and went on retreat during my own time in the pregnancy and postpartum period. My practice and my writing was deeply influenced by each of them: Nancy Bardacke, who developed the Mindfulness-Based Childbirth and Parenting program and wrote *Mindful Birthing*; Sarah Powers, who wrote *Insight Yoga*; and Richard Miller, who teaches iRest meditation. I encourage everyone to check out their wonderful work.

Thank you to the team at Postpartum Support International, for the work they do every day on behalf of the community of mothers with PMADs, for educating me, and for welcoming me to present at your conference, enabling me to see that this topic was interesting and valuable to more people than just me.

Thank you to all of my therapy clients, yoga students, and moms circle participants for being my greatest teachers. I feel honored and grateful that I get to spend my days listening, learning, witnessing, supporting, and connecting with you.

Thank you to my circle of friends who supported me through two pregnancies and the writing of this book—who cooked me meals, shared their own stories, loved me through my messiest days. I can't name you all here, but please know that I love you. Special thanks to Leah Chalofsky, my dearest, who was right there as my first baby entered the room. Thank you for being there through all my ups and downs and sharing yours with me since we were teenagers. Naomi Rudolph, thank you for bringing so much joy and sisterhood in those early days with our babies. Liora Kahn, thank you for always making me feel like I can just be myself. Thank you to the beloved women in my Rosh Chodesh group, who encouraged me to follow my heart and take time away to write, who inspire me as mothers and women. Special thanks to Miranda Weintraub, Ariel Berson, and Tali Ziv, for picking up my kids or hosting them for playdates when I was working late or running late. You all teach me every day that it really does take a village.

Thank you to my beloved colleagues—or, rather, friends that I work with—for teaching me, inspiring me, listening to me complain, and giving me confidence. With all of you in my life, these past few years in the East Bay have been the richest years I've had as a therapist. Thanks to the amazing community of practitioners at Rockridge Wellness Center. Thanks to Ariel Trost, Lynn Tracy, Maria-Christina Stewart, and Elizabeth Burns Kramer, for your stimulating, supportive, and meaningful collaboration and consultation. Thank you to Lee Safran for inspiring me to think more about the concept of maternal ambivalence and to the therapists in the maternal ambivalence study group.

Thank you to my friends and colleagues who read through the early drafts of this book to give me feedback: Cathy Berman, Elizabeth Burns Kramer, Leah Chalofsky, Antonia Fokken, Ayelet Kreiger, Dana Neufeld, Maria-Christina Stewart, and Melissa Whippo. Thank you for all your kind words, but even more for your willingness to give critical feedback.

Thank you especially to Elizabeth Burns Kramer, for your texts, your talks and walks, your advice, and your loving sense of humor. You have been the most gracious cheerleader around this book, as a colleague, and as a dear friend. I feel so incredibly lucky and grateful to have you in my life and across the hall.

Thank you to the childcare providers and teachers who are part of my children's community. Working parents don't do it on our own: we rely on people who make it their life's work to love our kids all day. Thank you especially to Angela Castro and Rosa-Maria Parraga.

Thanks to my family. To my parents, Emily and Marc Tipermas; my in-laws, Tess and Bruce Wilkoff; my aunt-in-law, Sheri Neufeld; and my sisters, Jane Tipermas and Katie Stull—thank you all for supporting and loving all of us through the births of both our kids and through this project. Dana Neufeld, my sister-in-law, this book owes a lot to your brainstorming help, your editing, and your deep insight. Special thanks to my mom for compromising your sleep and accompanying me and Ayelet on our crazy mindfulness retreat when she was just six months old.

Most of all, thank you to my husband, David, for all the solo parenting you did while I worked on this book, for cooking me countless meals so that I didn't have to pause in my writing, and for encouraging me and cheering me on. Thank you for helping me through our darkest times and for being an amazing love and father. Thank you to my daughters, Noa and Ayelet, who let me go write even when they wanted me all to themselves, who wrote me cards, sang me songs, and love me so unconditionally. I love you both to the moon and back. I'm so lucky to be your mom.

INDEX

abhinivesha, 113
acceptance and change,
    balancing, 47–49
Acceptance and
    Commitment
    Therapy (ACT), 36
activation, 107
advice, unsolicited, 163–
    64, 165
affirmations, 77
ahimsa, 186, 232
alternate nostril breathing,
    205
ambivalence, 123–25, 126
anger, 119–22
antidepressants, 37–39
anxiety. *See also* PMADs
    activation and, 107–8
    loss and, 143
    moving with, 108–9
    perinatal, 29–30
aparigraha, 176
appetite, 52–53
asanas (poses). *See also*
    individual poses
    with baby, 86
    mastery of, 229
    meaning of, 43, 48
    as metaphors, 78–79
asmita, 169
Austin, Jane, 14, 83, 88,
    115, 132
avidya, 157

baby
    active poses with, 86
    bonding with, 87–89
    breathing with, 86
    compassion for, 139
    crying, 137–39, 186
    optimizing, 175–76
    sleeping, 206–7
    walking back and forth
        with, 140–42
baby blues, 25–26

backbend, seated or
    standing basic, 198
bee breath, 204–5
beginner's mind, 233–37
belly
    breathing, 75–76
    soft, 173–74
bhakti yoga, 44
bipolar disorder, 29
birth
    "natural," 167–68
    plan, 65, 131
blame, 62–63, 119
body image, 171–74, 215,
    216
body scan, 208–9
bonding, 87–89
breastfeeding, 218–20
breath cycle awareness,
    82–83
breathing
    alternate nostril, 205
    with baby, 86
    bee, 204–5
    belly, 75–76
    easy rhythmic, 203
    importance of, 74–75
    "just this inhale," 111
    observing, 75
butterfly pose, 176–77

cat/cow, 165–66
chair pose, 179–80
change
    balancing acceptance
        and, 47–49
    difficulty of, 90–91
chest stretch, standing, 198
child's pose, 200–201
choice, 230–32
cognitive behavioral
    therapy (CBT), 36,
    45, 126
comparisons, 154–56
compassion

for baby, 139
    meaning of, 147
    practicing, 144–45, 164
    self-, 147–49, 151, 172
corpse pose. *See* savasana
crying, 103–4, 137–39, 186

death, thoughts about,
    134–36
depression. *See also*
    PMADs
    darkest thoughts of,
        134–36
    etymology of, 46, 144
    loss and, 143
    perinatal, 26, 28–29
    postpartum, 26
    range of, 29
    sadness vs., 28
    symptoms of, 28–29
    treatment for, 36–40
dialectical behavior therapy
    (DBT), 36, 59
discipline, 52
discomfort, 115
downward-facing dog pose,
    223–24
dukha, 46

easy seated pose, 197
eating
    disorders, 32–33
    mindful, 216–17
ego, noticing, 169
emotional regulation,
    46–47, 120
emotions. *See* feelings
equanimity, cultivating,
    130–32
exercise, 221–22
exhaustion, 199–200

fatigue, 199–200
fear, 107, 113, 127
feeding meditation, 220

feelings
  identifying, 102
  opposite, 123–25
  resisting, 100–101
  sitting with, 100
  thoughts vs., 102
  welcoming, 100, 101–2, 125
"fight, flight, or freeze" response, 107
flying cat pose, 194–95
food struggles, 214–17
fortune-telling, 110
forward fold, standing, 187–88
future-tripping, 110

gratitude, 126
grief, 143–45

hatha yoga, 44
heart-openers, 196–98
help, asking for, 94–98
hypervigilance, 230
hypomania, 29

interoception, 179–80
Iyengar, B. K. S., 196

jnana yoga, 44
journaling, mindful, 64
judging, 160–62, 215
"juicy hips," 83

karma yoga, 44
karuna, 147
keep-ups, 115–18
kleshas, 113
koshas, 211

legs up the wall, 201–2
letting go, 164, 183
light within, 88–89
lion's breath, 122

mania, 29
manifesting, 126
massage, 149–50
mastery, 228, 229

maternal instincts, lack of, 233
medications, 37–39
meditation
  anxiety and, 72–73
  basic, 71
  benefits of, 72
  feeding, 220
  myths about, 70
  opposite emotions, 125
  preoccupations and, 113–14
  soft-belly, 173–74
  sound, 212–13
  walking, 141–42
  yoga nidra, 199
  on your changing body, 173
  zooming, 170
mindfulness
  eating and, 216–17
  journaling and, 64
  marketing of, 42
  meaning of, 190
  moving with, 104–6
  pregnancy and, 85
  present moment focus, 190–91
  rephrasing and, 158–59
  therapy and, 36–37
motherhood
  challenges of, 9–10, 18–19, 24–25, 34–35, 147, 189–90
  myths about, 17, 24, 160
  "natural," 167–69
mountain pose, 91–92, 93

nadi shodana, 205
natural mandate, 167–69
nausea, 13–15
neck stretch, 232
negative thoughts, automatic, 157–59, 160
nonjudging, 161–62, 215

object permanence, 212

OCD (obsessive-compulsive disorder), 30–31
OM, chanting, 203–4
opposite action, taking, 59–60

pain, 115, 127, 192–94
Patanjali, 48, 88, 156, 203
permission, giving yourself, 151–53
plank pose, 224–25
planning, 65–69, 130–31
pleasure, importance of, 81
PMADs (perinatal mood and anxiety disorders)
  baby blues vs., 25–26
  healing from, 21, 41
  meaning of, 10
  plan for, 65–68
  prevalence of, 10, 26
  risk factors for, 33–35
  subtypes of, 28–33
  symptoms of, 26, 27–28
  treatment for, 35–40
poses. See asanas
positive thinking, 126
posture, 196–98
prana, 74
pranayama, 74, 203
pratyahara, 164–66, 204, 212
pregnancy
  challenges of, 9, 18, 24–25, 147, 189–90
  discomfort during, 115
  mindfulness and, 85
  preoccupations, 112–14
  present moment focus, 190–91
psychodynamic therapy, 36
psychosis, 33
PTSD (post-traumatic stress disorder), 31–32

rage, 119–22
rainbow arms, 197